MW00438205

"I was blessed enough nutrition…the main ing hockey career. This bc athlete to take control of their dream so at the end of the day you can say you did everything you could do to be the best you can be."

~ Riley Cote, Former left winger for the Philadelphia Flyers
and currently the Assistant Coach of their minor league team,
the Lehigh Valley Phantoms

Body Balance Empowering Performance by Deborah Dittner is a great resource for all you athletes out there. Deborah gives you all the information you need to properly fuel your body for optimal performance on and off the playing field. You will find great recipes for natural rehydrating drinks so you can avoid the unhealthy sport's drinks on the market and give your body what it needs during and after intense exercise. I know you will be coming back to this guide again and again to learn all about the power of nutrition. Enjoy!

~ Elizabeth W Boham MD, MS, RD, UltraWellness Center, Lenox,
MA

"Deb understands that nutrition isn't just about improving your athletic performance but how it can improve your overall life. Deb's approach is professional and adjusts well to each person's nutritional needs."

~ Kyle Flanagan, St. Lawrence University graduate
BA in Performance and Communication Arts
St Lawrence University Division I Hockey 2009-2013
2012 ECAC Third Team
2013 Hobey Baker Finalist. NCAA DIV I First team All-American
ECAC First Team
Signed NHL contract with the Philadelphia Flyers
2013-2014 Played for the Adirondack Phantoms of the AHL
2014-2015 playing with MODO Hockey of the Swedish Elite League

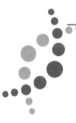

"If we could give every individual the right amount of nourishment and exercise, not too little and not too much, we would have found the safest way to health."
~ **Hippocrates**

"Deborah has been an excellent resource for our younger players. You'll find in her book that she is willing to be a resource for you! Deb's book contains some very valuable information to help improve you overall health and fitness."
~ Jim McCrossin, MS ATC, CSCS, PES, CES Head Athletic Trainer and Strength and Conditioning Coach for the Philadelphia Flyers

"An easy read that allows all levels of athletes to relate to, enabling them to take ownership in the simplicity of eating healthy, towards better performance in sports and their daily life"
~ Sean Flanagan, Assistant Hockey Coach, Hobart College, Geneva, NY.
St. Lawrence University Graduate with a BS in History and minor in Sport Studies and Exercise Sciences and a Master's in Education. Played Division I Hockey at St. Lawrence University

"Coming from a traditional education in healthcare, Deborah has diversified her knowledge base and practice to include clinical nutrition and a holistic approach to health and wellness. A gifted practitioner blending traditional and alternative medicine to create lifestyles that compliment and improve daily living for her patients. A true blessing to our practice and our patients."
~ Kenneth Sullivan-Bol, DC, Chiropractic Physician Orthopedics and Sports Medicine

SHIRES✸PRESS

P.O. Box 2200
4869 Main Street
Manchester Center, VT 05255
www.northshire.com

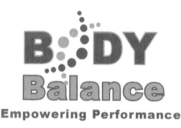

Empowering Performance

ISBN: 978-1-60571-226-0

Cover photo: Fred Troilo • Fred Troilo Photography • www.fredtroilo.com

NORTHSHIRE BOOKSTORE
Building Community, One Book at a Time
*A family-owned, independent bookstore in
Manchester Ctr., VT, since 1976 and Saratoga Springs, NY since 2013.
We are committed to excellence in bookselling.
The Northshire Bookstore's mission is to serve as a resource for
information, ideas, and entertainment while honoring the needs of
customers, staff, and community.*

Printed in the United States of America

To Jimmy
In Health and
Happiness !
Be Well
Deb

B🔵DY
Balance

Empowering Performance

Deborah Dittner
FNP-C, RMT, CHHC, AADP

"I hope to provide you, the reader, the athlete, the coach, the parent, the team, the athletic trainer, and the weekend warrior, with information necessary to make the best educated decisions on lifestyle changes for a healthier, more balanced you."

~ Deborah Dittner

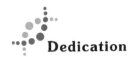# Dedication

To my three children Krissa, Misha, and Kat who have inspired me throughout their lives filled with sport and determination. It has been my greatest privilege being your mom. I love you always.

To those women and men I have worked with over the years providing me the platform to continue to search for ways to improve their health and wellness through balance.

To my students who have taught me a few things over time.

To "Coach" Sandra White, East Lyme High School, East Lyme, CT for providing me with inspiration and guidance.

To Lesley Waters, the best massage therapist and much appreciated editor of this book that was so passionately created. Your devoted time and energy and understanding will always be cherished.

To Riley Cote, Assistant Coach of the Lehigh Valley Phantoms (previously known as the Adirondack Phantoms), and the Lehigh Valley Phantoms team for their devotion, search for knowledge, and excellence in athleticism. May you always keep the passion in your hearts and the desire to fulfill your dreams.

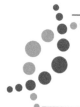

"I encourage you to recognize and appreciate all that inspires you to feel empowered."

~ **Deborah Dittner**

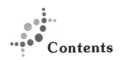

Contents

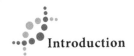

Introduction

Body Balance Empowering Performance is the passionate work I have dedicated my career towards. I hope to provide you, the reader, the athlete, the coach, the parent, the team, the athletic trainer, and the weekend warrior, with information necessary to make the best educated decisions on lifestyle changes for a healthier, more balanced you. There's a lot of information out there, some contradictory, seemingly produced daily! I'm here to help you sort through that ever-changing information and determine what works best for you, the individual. I feel it's important to present the significance of eating clean and balancing the body for all athletes and specifically, the professional hockey player. The intention of this book is to empower each and every athlete to take control of their dream (to play professionally) so at the end of the day you can say "I did everything I could do to be the best I can be." I also want to provide the needed information for you to make very educated decisions when it comes to the fuel you put into your body, your temple, and for you to dig deep into looking at your life style, what you are eating, and if it's working for you or against you.

Deborah Dittner is a Family Nurse Practitioner, Reiki Master Teacher and Certified Holistic Health Counselor. As a high school student I played three sports: tennis, basketball (co-captain, high rebounder, MVP) and track and field (co-captain, 100 yard, third leg of the 400 yard relay and high jump with a number of records). I attended Western Connecticut State University majoring in nursing as the nurturing part of me was in high gear. While in college, I began to referee basketball and volleyball and years later became certified to coach on the high school level. Long distance running led to often being in the top 3 of my age group in local road races. As my children grew, sports were a huge part of their lives as well, varying from volleyball, basketball, soccer, and softball, and all coached by mom at one time or another. They have continued their athletic quests running marathons, playing ice hockey and rugby. During these years and reading many books, articles, attending conferences, and through my personal research, I passionately spoke about the health benefits of clean eating and cooking, the importance of sleep, physical movement, social life, education and career, creativity, stress management, and self-care, not just for individual clients but for all athletes alike.

Sharing information about all the things that I love about health is my passion. Health is a blending of many things; the food we eat, the thoughts we think, the relationships we nurture, the exercise we provide for our body, the profession and pastimes we devote ourselves to, and the passionate commitment of our souls. All of these things take love, dedication, and compassion to balance our health and happiness. What motivates me to continue to do what I do best are those who I have guided to a better life from athletes to diabetics to obese people to those who want to live to a ripe old age with as minimal of problems as possible. Our nutrition, our eating clean, the wholesome foods that we put into our body is what motivates me to educate each and every one of you. When I talk about eating clean, a part of me comes out that is pure enthusiasm. I've instilled into my children that eating clean is a way of life and our kitchens are our wellness centers. Where there is food, there's life. It's what carries us on to bigger and better, and more fulfilled lives.

I was asked at a Wellness Committee Meeting for a corporation to name two good foods and two not-so-good foods. My two favorites which I also consider "super foods" would be kale and hemp seeds. As you continue to read throughout this book, you will see many references to both of these so I'll save the "whys" for then. The two not-so-good would be those processed and highly refined foods and sugar. I'll refer to these later on as well. It's talking with groups like the Wellness Committee, professional hockey players, and you that continue my devotion to educate towards a balanced body.

Creating balance in our lives is a step by step process that simply doesn't happen overnight. This process needs to be developed and nurtured. By following your passion, being true to yourself, and working hard toward your goals will bring you to that reality.

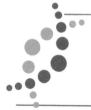

"My two favorite 'good foods,' which I also consider super foods would be kale and hemp seeds."
~ **Deborah Dittner**

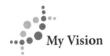 **My Vision**

The mission here is quite simple. My vision is to help empower all people. Athlete or not, this book will help you look at things a bit differently and help guide you along in your journey no matter what it might be. My goal is to explain nutrition in the simplest way using basic common sense so you will have the knowledge to consciously choose foods wisely. Taking control of your health and your destiny is a key part of your spiritual journey. Reconnecting with all the powerful foods that Mother Nature has to offer is the perfect way to start.

As you read about what I whole-heartedly believe in, you may wonder why there is an emphasis on professional ice hockey. Over the years, my youngest daughter and I had watched our local AHL team develop and followed their progress. The Adirondack Phantoms, now the Lehigh Valley Phantoms, was our home team and I had the pleasure of working with a few of the players individually. Food journals led to the encouragement of clean eating and how the body is your temple. Grocery store tours and the importance of reading a label, recipes for pre- and post-game meals, ways to manage sleep and stress and travel were amongst the numerous topics of discussion. Through this work, I have found that nutrition needs to come more to the foreground of what is necessary to make a professional athlete.

New Year's Eve 2013, a dear friend and colleague sent an Instagram message which I didn't read until the morning on New Year's Day. It reads:

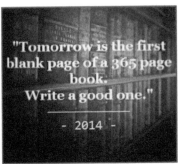

"Tomorrow is the first blank page of a 365 page book. Write a good one."

- 2014 -

Well …that got me thinking and since then, I have taken that blank page and have turned it in to what I believe is needed to help the athlete and all individuals alike bring more balance into their lives for health and wellness.

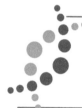

"The food you eat can be either the safest and most powerful form of medicine or the slowest form of poison."

~ **Ann Wigmore**

Part One

Your Body. Your Temple.

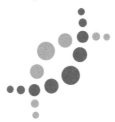

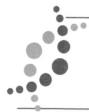

"Processed foods were not introduced into the human diet until the start of the 20th century."

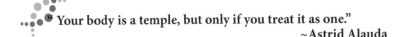 **Your body is a temple, but only if you treat it as one."**
~Astrid Alauda

If you ask any athlete what their ultimate goal is, it's surely to attain the highest level possible in any given sport and of course to win at each level. Most athletes are very driven with a direct focus on doing whatever it takes to reach these goals. But competitive sports aren't something new. In fact they have been a part of different countries and cultures for thousands of years. The first recorded ancient Olympics in Olympia, Greece games date back before 776 BC. Since the competitiveness in man has not changed over time, I think it's fair to say these athletes trained hard, practiced hard and had one goal in mind, and that was to win. But what would an athlete have used as fuel to meet the energy needs for such a demanding competition?

Well I can assure you that there were no "sports drinks", "endurance gels" or any "protein bars" back then. Sports performance supplements/processed foods were clearly not options for these athletes. To put everything in perspective, all processed foods were not introduced into the human diet until the start of the 20th century. That's only in the last 115 years or so ago, when you compare it to the total timeline of how long man has been walking this planet. Now processed foods and sports performance supplements have become huge business, taking over the food industry. More and more nutrient depleted foods are finding their way into grocery stores, sporting good stores and convenience stores. We have become so disconnected from what's real and what's not.

The human being is a perfectly orchestrated machine designed to eat all the great nutrient dense food sources that God has put on this green earth such as vegetables, fruits, seeds, nuts and wild and grass-fed lean animal sources. We are not designed to eat foods stripped of its nutrition in a factory, rearranged and added back into an extremely high sugar/high sodium product that tastes great and has very limited nutritional value. No, these calories are cheap because they are cheap. Marketing is everything for these companies. It doesn't matter if your product is good or not, healthy or not but if you make people believe it is, then you sell a ton of product and you control the market. And that's exactly what's happened. Just follow the money $. These companies' products are cheap, nutrient-depleted, and use refined, genetically modified corn syrups/sugars as their main ingredients. They also include artificial electrolytes and ascorbic acid as vitamin C. It becomes a sports drink.

You can sell anything to anyone as long as you make them a believer in what you are selling and that's simply marketing.

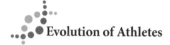

Evolution of Athletes

The sports industry has become an incredibly huge business. From basically nothing, the ancient Olympians competed for their countries and for personal pride almost three thousand years ago to gladiators fighting to the death in the famous Coliseum in Rome to present day professionals making millions of dollars a year. Athletes are bigger, faster and stronger than they have ever been. They train harder and more specific to their individual sports than they ever have. Yet most athletes never truly understand the most important variable in the process of becoming an elite athlete and that's nutrition. We have complicated a very simple concept with biased science so that big business can sell you more of their cheap, processed and dead foods. Today's athletes, like previous athletes, are constantly seeking any edge to maximize performance, however most athletes are sincerely wrong when it comes to diet, nutrition and preparing for competition. The problem is these man-made manufactured products really don't work. They are packed with empty calories and highly-heated protein concentrates but are not the answer for real sustainable energy. We must reconnect with our roots and consume a diet of mainly plant based whole foods to get that sustainable energy that all people including athletes need.

You might be skeptical that there is no way you can compete at the highest level of competition on whole foods. The formula remains the same whether you are just looking to become healthier or if you plan on fueling up as an elite athlete. Since athletes clearly burn more calories and need sustainable energy to train, compete and recover, they simply need to increase their caloric intake with more plant based whole foods. While each individual is different, listening to your body is key. Learning and knowing your body is essential for optimum performance. Once you reconnect with your inner being and understand how real whole foods work in the human body, you will be fully empowered to take your God given ability to the highest level possible.

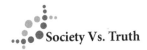# Society Vs. Truth

We used to think the earth was flat. Science once told us that. Science has helped us come a long way, but it has also become completely profit driven and biased, all depending on who is funding the "study." Big business profits off science because they can prove whatever they want. Always look into who is funding the study and who is profiting off the science of it. The problem lies in the hands of reductionist science. If you are a reductionist, you would believe that everything in the world can be understood if you understand all of its parts. On the other hand a wholist believes that the "whole" can be greater than the sum of its parts. This debate has been going on since the start of time and even though reductionist science has given us some major breakthroughs in the past several centuries, this type of science will never fully be able to explain something as simple as how eating an apple digests, assimilates and nourishes the body.

Much like all whole foods, a simple apple is made up of thousands of compounds and antioxidants that all work synergistically together in the body. With all these chemical reactions taking place in your body, there is no way of ever calculating the specific influence of each chemical as there is an infinite number of possible biological consequences. While a wholistic approach understands everything as a whole, it acknowledges that eating whole foods nourishes and fuels the body much more efficiently than separate compounds individually ever will.

Please understand that wholism does not oppose reductionism but rather encompasses it, just as each whole encompasses its parts. This becomes a breeding ground for profit driven big business that take advantage of selling and marketing separate parts of foods such as vitamin C, omega fatty acids and different types of protein. All end up being heavily processed and let's face it, they don't work the same in the human body. As a society we have become very naive in believing everything we are told and everything we see on TV. We have become disconnected from the natural world and unfortunately there is a price to pay. Disease has reached epidemic levels as well as obesity and mental illness. The most fundamental part of the human race, basic nutrition, has been completely ignored and overlooked as if it has no value on human health or performance.

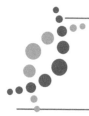

Becoming Empowered

As an athlete looks at their career, they constantly seek different ways to become the best they can be. And rightfully so, that's the whole point isn't it? It's tempting to think that nutrition "products" could give athletes the edge they desire, but it's simply marketing. Nothing replaces simple, healthy, whole foods. Nutrition is the cornerstone of health, who we are and what we can ultimately achieve. As an athlete, proper nutrition can help with prevention of injury, increased performance, recovery, focus and healing. Learning to respect and listen to your body is a key component to fully maximizing the power of nutrition. Let's face it, we are all different. No two people or athletes are the same. While one whole food might be great for one individual, it might not be for another.

This is the reason I decided to write this book, to empower you, the athlete and the non-athlete to be accountable and to make conscious decisions that will lead to optimum health and maximized performance. Mother Nature has blessed us with thousands of nutrient dense plants and foods so explore the many options that are readily available at your local health food store. It is the age of information so do yourself a favor and get on google and read up on anything that sparks your interest. Be sure to read both sides of the story and then create your own personal opinion based on the facts. Try to make the most sense of what's real and what's not and if it's going to work for you. Reconnecting with the natural world and the powerful whole foods it offers, is the ideal way to fuel up and is the only way to achieve the sustainable energy we are all looking for. The power ultimately lies in your hands. We don't need to complicate this subject. Eating natural, whole foods worked for thousands of years and it still works today.

"Why is obesity the norm these days and so accepted? Because society tells us it's normal."

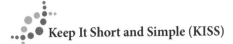 **Keep It Short and Simple (KISS)**

How did we ever become so disconnected with our inner beings and the natural world? How come everything these days seems so complicated? From the water we drink to the food we eat to the way we exercise. There are all kinds of contradicting opinions and information around. I'm telling you from personal experience and everything I've learned that the most basic fundamentals for human survival really couldn't be simpler. However, to understand the simplicity of these daily fundamentals, we must open up our minds and change the way we think. We have all been programmed to think a certain way based on what society wants us to believe. Why is obesity the norm these days and so accepted? Because society tells us it's normal.

The simple fix for this would be to cram in plant based whole foods and cram out all the toxic processed and chemically infused man-made foods. Your body would naturally be forced to lose weight based on sheer physics. Instead it is normal in the western world to seek all kinds of health care professionals, try all kinds of fad diets and buy the latest weight loss supplements on the market. Following the money trail usually helps explain who is profiting from misinformation and why science can be so confusing at times. The sad part is most people can't see the forest through the trees. The solution to this madness is getting back to basics, keeping it simple, and to just use a little God given common sense.

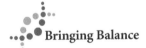 **Bringing Balance**

There is no magic pill to optimum health. It's a way of life. Reconnecting to the natural world is essential in becoming a conscious being. Simplifying your diet based on logic and common sense is not a new idea, but an important one. The actual "nutrition" in food is a variable that is loosely talked about and has become extremely complicated and often ignored. While there are more variables to optimum health than just diet and nutrition, it remains the largest variable in a holistic approach, which strongly endorses prevention.

The dietary approach in this book is by no means pushing a specific and limited diet like becoming vegetarian, vegan, a raw foodie or paleo.

While the words vegetarian and vegan sound extremely healthy to most people there are such thing as junk food vegetarians and vegans who consume many denatured processed foods as a primary source of their diet. Hell, Oreos are vegan! The point I'm making is, by identifying the way you eat by a word that limits you to not eating fish or meat doesn't mean you are as healthy as you could be.

Raw foodies consume a diet of 100% raw foods. While I agree with the concept of maximizing nutrition through raw whole foods, and incorporating them, there must be balance maintained in the body. Raw foods are cold or (yin) to the body according to Chinese medicine. Too much cold throws off your body's balance and creates a vulnerable environment. Consuming some lightly cooked or steamed whole foods have a warming or (yang) effect on your body and help to regain balance. A good example of this is during cold and flu season. I do believe if you maintain proper balance in your body with nutrition and stress management, you can avoid getting a cold or the flu, however, there are times when your body gets run down and you can get sick.

Moms are known to make soothing soup broth and possibly brew some hot herbal teas. These help bring warmth and balance to the body and are really low stress on the digestive track helping you get well sooner. Eating raw and cooling foods during this time would slow down the healing process because it puts your body more off balance. Paleo is a relatively new fad diet with an age old approach. Paleo is a diet of cavemen that consists of high animal protein, no grains or legumes. Even though I do agree with hunter/gatherer mentality as there is no denying we are all animals on quest for survival, they exclude some valuable whole foods that help with sustained energy. Adding some whole grains and legumes can be very helpful to maintaining balance and an ideal body weight.

Protein is important but not any more important than the rest of the equation. We need protein but there are plenty of plant based food sources that contain high levels of protein. I don't believe we need as much animal protein as the Paleo diet recommends and as the western world says we do. Choose clean animal protein sources like grass fed/ free range beef and pasture raised chickens and low mercury wild fish like salmon. Limit your animal protein intake to a logical percentage of your diet. Consuming a diet of around 5% clean properly raised animal protein is ideal and realistic.

To best summarize the type of diet I am promoting to help create balance in the body and increase performance on all levels is to get back to basics and our roots. We were intended to eat a wide array of nutrient rich whole foods that are grown naturally, not heavily sprayed or genetically modified, processed foods that offer nothing but empty calories to the body. Wild game and properly farmed animal protein sources not only offer healthy protein and cleaner nutrition, they help encourage a healthier environment by lowering the carbon footprint. Factory farms are inhumane and breed and raise extremely polluted animals. My goal is to help you become empowered, so you can consciously make the best decisions in regards to choosing your fuel.

Keep it fresh. Get creative and experience the many different whole foods that the natural world has to offer. They are all loaded with nutrition. Individually we are all a bit different; there is no one universal diet that is fool proof. Rely on local climate and agricultural practices. Certain foods that grow in the Mediterranean surely wouldn't be growing in Canada. However, the formula remains the same no matter where you are on the planet. A diet rich in whole foods, limited and clean animal protein, plus stress management all equates to optimum health and performance. On the other hand, a western diet, a diet high in fat, rich in processed foods, dairy products, refined sugars and extremely high amounts of animal protein only equate to an acidic, inflamed, and imbalanced body leading to sickness and lower energy and performance. The western diet's end results are western diseases such as obesity, diabetes, heart disease and numerous forms of cancer.

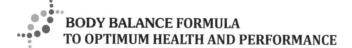

BODY BALANCE FORMULA
TO OPTIMUM HEALTH AND PERFORMANCE

☑ **Represents variables that have positive impacts on enhancing health and performance**

☑ Stay hydrated with pure water
☑ Increase whole foods (vegetables, fruits, seeds, nuts whole grains, legumes)
☑ Increase RAW whole foods (foods in their natural state-such as salads, fruit, seeds, nuts)
☑ Choose organic foods whenever possible
☑ Limited high quality fish and meat
☑ Limited high quality plant base oils
☑ Maintain a balanced body (pH level)
☑ Proper rest and recovery
☑ More natural fruit sugars and electrolytes should be consumed as work load and exercise levels increase

☒ **Represents variables that have negative impacts on enhancing health and performance**

☒ Avoid and limit processed foods
☒ Avoid and limit refined sugars
☒ Avoid and limit dairy products
☒ Avoid and limit genetically modified ingredients (GMOs)
☒ Avoid and limit conventionally farmed meat
☒ Avoid and limit farm raised fish
☒ Avoid and limit stress
☒ Avoid and limit the consumption of alcohol

The simple formula here is to focus on and increase the ☑ in your daily routine and consciously avoid and minimize the ☒. By cramming out the foods that are acidic, inflammatory and harmful to the body's balance, you will then in turn cram in alkaline forming, anti inflammatory, nutrient rich whole foods which help maximize a balanced and healthy body.

So it looks like this.

☑ = increased + health and performance
☒ = decreased - health and performance

☑ + ☑ = health and Performance level +2
☑ + ☑ + ☑ = health and performance level +3
☑ + ☑ + ☑ + ☑ = health and performance
      level +4 and so on…

☒ + ☒ = health and performance level - 2
☒ + ☒ + ☒ = health and performance level - 3
☒ + ☒ + ☒ + ☒ = health and performance
      level - 4 and so on…

☑ + ☒ = health and performance level 0
☑ + ☑ + ☒ = health and performance level + 1
☑ + ☑ + ☑ + ☒ = health and performance
      level + 2
☑ + ☑ + ☒ + ☒ = health and performance level 0

Everything you do in life will either work for you or work against you, either improves health and performance or decreases it. In this example the variables with the ☑, will not only help bring balance to the body which promotes general health, healing and focus, it helps the body to sustain maximum performance. The variables with the ☒, work against the body creating an acidic environment, an imbalanced body and decreases sustained energy and performance.

"Everything you do in life will either work for you or work against you, either improves health and performance or decreases it."

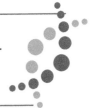

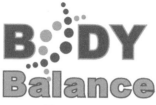

Formula

+5 — INCREASED PERFORMANCE

+4

+3

+2

☑ +1

0 — AVERAGE PERFORMANCE

☒ -1

-2

-3

-4

DECREASED PERFORMANCE
-5

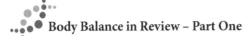 **Body Balance in Review – Part One**

☑ Take care of the temple and the temple will take care of you…physically, mentally and emotionally. As individuals, you need to find that balance of eating clean, physical movement, sleep, and overall self-care.

☑ The progression of athleticism from ancient Olympians to today's multi-million dollar contracts still has one very important aspect to the goals and that is a high quality, whole foods diet to provide the necessary energy for performance.

☑ Marketing is big business. Millions of dollars goes into the selling of supplements, protein powders, sports drinks and more. Looking at the truth (and ingredients) behind these products is to be researched and understood.

☑ Nutrition is the cornerstone of health. Listen to your body. Make the most of your God given talents and take control of your life.

☑ Creating balance in your body through a diet rich in whole, nutrient dense foods combined with lifestyle changes will lead to optimum health and performance.

"As individuals, you need to find that balance of eating clean, physical movement, sleep, and overall self-care."

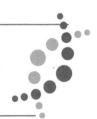

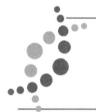

*"Stress creates an acidic environment
in the body that leads to imbalances
that can cause medical issues."*

Part Two

Body Basics

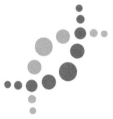

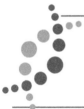

"For an athlete, exercise and physical stress are absolutely necessary for training and getting into proper condition to compete at the highest level."

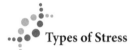# The Effect of Stress

Stress is inevitable and has become rampant in today's society whether you're an athlete or not. Day-in and day-out stress creates an acidic environment in the body that leads to imbalances that can cause medical issues. Chronic stress elevates cortisol levels (the stress hormone), causes an increase in insulin and inflammation which can create excess fat specifically around the middle, adds to insulin resistance, may lead to weight gain, and plays a large role in emotions. An increase in stress hormones can increase cravings and overeating, and cause hormone imbalances. Stress reduction can help lower blood pressure, cholesterol levels, and overall inflammation.

Types of Stress

Most people think of stress as that feeling when you are pressured to get something done, yet it is much deeper than that. Today's stressors are much different and have become much more complex than they were back in the day. In the world today, the obvious daily stressors would include finances, job deadlines and security, traffic, kids and much more. Work is also stress. Otherwise it would be called "fun" or a "vacation." Basic survival, such as finding food and maintaining shelter, would be the main stressors dealt with thousands of years ago. One huge stressor most people do not acknowledge is digestive stress. The amount of work your digestive system requires to break down foods and ultimately absorb the nutrients is enormous. If you have embraced the standard western diet of refined, processed, fat and denatured foods (**ENERGY** -), your digestive track is surely working overtime and causing much unneeded stress on the body. The simple way to manage this type of stress would be to adopt a mainly whole food diet of fresh vegetables, fruits, nuts, seeds, whole grains (**ENERGY** +) and limited high quality animal protein. These foods are digested much easier, reducing the amount of work your body needs to put forth to retrieve the nutrition it needs. Digestive stress is an extremely manageable stress that can change the way you feel and the way you live your life. Physical stress would include anything from working a labor job such as construction to landscaping around the house to any form of exercise.

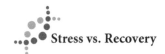 **Stress vs. Recovery**

For an athlete, exercise and physical stress are absolutely necessary for training and getting into proper condition to compete at the highest level. Breaking down muscle tissue is the only way to stimulate the regeneration of new cells. Once any form of exercise, practice or game is complete, the recovery process immediately begins. This means minimizing or removing any unnecessary stressors as this is wasted energy. The more stress you can manage, the more energy your body will have to repair and recover. It's that simple. Everything you do from the time you complete your exercise/training regimen is preparing you to be as fresh as you can be for the following practice or game. Again, digestive stress tops the list as a stress that can be easily managed by consuming more whole foods (**ENERGY +**) for two reasons. The first is obvious, the less work your body requires to break down food for energy, the better. Second, you will be fueling up with nutrient rich foods therefore regenerating the cells much quicker.

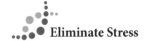 **Eliminate Stress**

☑ **Breath work** – Breathing techniques have been shown to reduce stress and anxiety, boost the immune system, lower blood pressure, improve concentration and focus, remove toxins, and improve energy production. Breathing techniques can be quite simple, take little time, can be done anywhere, and should be practiced everyday. Deep, slow, full breaths can correct the stress response by stimulating the rest and digest side of the nervous system. The vagus nerve goes through the diaphragm and moves with each deep breath creating relaxation. Sit comfortably and take five (5) good, deep breaths and then note how you feel.

An example of a breathing technique is as follows: Sit comfortably with your feet on the floor and hands resting comfortably in your lap. Close your mouth and inhale through your nose to a count of four (4). Hold your breath to the count of seven (7). Exhale fully through the mouth to the count of eight (8). Repeat this sequence three (3) more times for an entire cycle of four (4) breaths.

I recommend breath work on awakening, before bed, and any other time(s) throughout the day when stressed or anxious. Additional breathing techniques can be found at **www.drweil.com**

☑ **Calming Teas** – There are a variety of calming and soothing teas that can help eliminate stress. One of my favorites is a Calming Turmeric Tea which is also anti-inflammatory. It's a great tea after a hard game before bed. (see Recipes)

☑ **Emotional Freedom Technique (EFT)** – This practice aids in the release of emotions and pain. EFT is a form of energy therapy. Energy meridian points on the body are stimulated by tapping with your fingertips (approximately 7 times) while paying attention to the issue of concern. The intention of EFT is to rebalance the energy system. For more information go to **www.EFTUniverse.com** or Nick Ortner's book entitled *The Tapping Solution*.

☑ **Hot Bath or Sauna** – A hot bath with added bath salts and a relaxing therapeutic grade essential oil such as lavender helps your body to deeply relax. Epsom salts contains magnesium which reduces stress, anxiety, and depression and also creates relaxation.

☑ **Journaling** – Take a few minutes at the end of the day to write down those issues that may be bothering you. Don't evaluate your thoughts, just write them down. After you have flushed out the negativity, write down five (5) things that you are grateful for. Expressing gratitude ends journaling on a positive note and will allow for more restful sleep.

☑ **Laughter** – A good laugh with friends or watching a funny movie can have a huge effect on the stress response as laughter releases endorphins, natural stress busters, and also boosts the immune system.

☑ **Massage** – Massage is a useful calming and restorative therapy. Massage eases muscle tension and pain, improves digestion, improves mood, increases lymph flow, and accelerates the release of toxins from the body and lowers cortisol levels.

☑ **Meditation** – Mindful meditation reduces stress and negativity thus allowing the body to boost immunity which has been shown to decrease the number and severity of cold/flu symptoms by as much as 60%. Meditating on compassion has also been shown to help create a state of happiness. Meditation introduces a state of peacefulness and rest to the mind and body. There are a variety of ways to meditate from guided (on CDs) to walking labyrinths.

☑ **Reiki** – The healing art of Reiki addresses imbalances within your body to support your good health and well-being. This subtle form of energy therapy addresses both chronic and acute conditions, gently, and powerfully promoting balances among the body's systems and the normal regenerative processes of the body and mind. Reiki can complement other treatments by helping to reduce stress, calm the body for improved sleep, and reduce pain.

☑ **Therapeutic Grade Essential Oils** – Aromatherapy can improve mood, decrease stress and boost overall health. Essential oils used in stress relief are lavender, lemon, and basil to name a few (see Therapeutic Grade Essential Oils).

☑ **Yoga** – Yoga is not only a form of movement but it also aids in centering the body and creating calm. Regular yoga practice will help to boost your mind and decrease symptoms of depression. Numerous research studies have been done showing that yoga will lower stress hormone levels and increase the interruption of the anxiety neurotransmitter, GABA. One of the simplest and most effective yoga poses is a Bridge Pose as it opens the heart and lungs allowing oxygen to flow more freely.

"Sleep is the golden chain that binds health and our bodies together."

~ Thomas Dekker

Sleep

As a key part of the regenerative, aging and healing process, sleep is the cornerstone of recovery. Without adequate and proper sleep, the recovery process is negatively impacted and ultimately the consequence is sub-par performance. Research has shown that most adults need between seven and nine hours of quality sleep each night. Sleep is essential to maintain a healthy immune system, keeps you more alert, allows your body to make necessary repairs, improves memory and mental health, and decreases stress. A good night's sleep can also help to manage hunger, cravings, anxiety and mood. Poor or lack of sleep can lead to hormone imbalances which in turn can lead to more severe issues such as obesity, depression and diabetes. Whether you are an athlete or not, sleep ranks up there as one of the most important variables when it comes to general health, recovery and optimum performance.

When everything is in balance, you will experience a good night's sleep. When you sleep well, you will find balance in the remainder of your life. A magnesium rich diet (see Magnesium) consisting of plenty of leafy greens and nuts will aid in that balance.

Melatonin is a hormone produced in the body that is released naturally as exposure to sunlight decreases. It reduces alertness helping your body prepare for sleep. Limiting the exposure to light before bed may be extremely beneficial in your quality of sleep, especially if you are a person that has difficulty falling asleep. Develop a routine at bedtime approximately 30 minutes before you actually climb into bed as this will help to release the day's stress.

- ☒ Avoid the use of electronic devices (TV, computer, iPhone/iPad) at least one hour prior to bed time. These devices are stimulating and will not allow for a restful night's sleep.

- ☒ Avoid the use of stimulants such as alcohol, caffeine (avoid after 1 pm), sugar, and smoking.

- ☒ Avoid eating "bed time snacks" or going to bed on a full stomach. This can cause sleep issues and can create difficulty with fat burning.

☑ Take a warm bath with Epsom salts infused with a therapeutic grade essential oil to help induce sleep. Essential oils have been found to ease mental fatigue encouraging a more restful sleep. The oils are uplifting and calming, and can be put through a diffuser or directly inhaled. Essential oils of benefit are lavender (the mother of all essential oils), frankincense (the father of all essential oils), chamomile, clary sage, rose, orange, lemon, and basil just to name a few. (see Therapeutic Grade Essential Oils)

☑ A relaxing cup of non-caffeinated tea may help you drift off with more ease.

☑ Reading a book or magazine can also create relaxation.

☑ You may want to incorporate breathing techniques into your pre-sleep routine to quiet the mind. (see Stress/Breath Work)

☑ Relaxation yoga postures such as child's pose, legs up the wall, and corpse pose are very soothing.

☑ Calming, relaxing music or a sound machine of nature's effects can quiet a busy mind.

☑ Keep a regular schedule. Game days/nights make this difficult as you don't get home until 10:30 pm or later. Your mind may still be on the ice recreating a play or two, or you could be on the bus traveling home. It's hard to calm down. You might be staying in a hotel where sights and sounds make a restful night's sleep harder. In these situations, making the most of what is available is necessary. You may want to bring your own pillow, headphones for relaxing music, eye-darkening mask, and calming teas.

☑ Rise at the same time each morning, if possible.

☒ Limit exposure to light before bed.

Create a bedroom atmosphere that will enhance sleep:

- ☑ Sleep in a bed consisting of a good quality mattress and a firm pillow.

- ☑ Remove computers, television, or iPhone/Blackberry/Smart-phone.

- ☒ Block out all light by installing darkening shades and/or curtains.

- ☒ Maintain an average room temperature of 70 degrees (not too hot and not too cold).

Therapeutic Grade Essential Oils

I once again need to praise the power of Mother Nature as she has given us everything we need on this planet to thrive. Essential oils are the immune of the plant and are considered to be mankind's first medicine. Essential oils are the aromatic volatile oils coming from plants or plant parts (roots, leaves, flowers, seeds, resin, shrubs, and more) penetrating our cells to increase oxygen uptake, improve absorption of nutrients, enhance longevity, and help your body to detoxify. Usage includes applying topically, inhalation, or as a dietary supplement. All of the body's systems can benefit from using essential oils.

The athlete can benefit from the use of therapeutic grade essential oils as there are no side effects that pharmaceuticals have. Essential oils, "the life blood of the plant," can help in bringing balance to the body systems disrupted from travel (such as digestion, sleep), overuse injury and inflammation, and a variety of stressors.

Athletes are constantly dealing with bumps, bruises, and managing all sorts of acute injuries on a daily basis. Recovery is the name of the game and maximizing recovery time is necessary to consistently maintain an elite level of performance. Incorporating therapeutic grade essential oils into your lifestyle will bring nothing but positive results. Some of these oils have the power to help relieve inflammation and pain when applied topically with a carrier oil like jojoba, olive, hemp or coconut, or when applied neat (undiluted). Other essential oils, when inhaled, have positive psychological effects that can help manage stress, anxiety and even depression while other oils help you sleep. These oils are very potent and concentrated plant matter that can help anyone especially the athlete. See the list of therapeutic grade essential oils below and their functions. Note that many specific oils can be used for many different conditions.

☑ Inflammation:

Clove
Copaiba
Lavender
Melaleuca Alternifolia (tea tree)
Nutmeg
Peppermint
Roman Chamomile
Thyme
Wintergreen

☑ Sleep:

Cedarwood
Grapefruit
Lavender
Marjoram
Orange
Roman Chamomile
Sandalwood
Valerian
Vetiver

☑ Digestion:

Anise
Clove
Fennel
Ginger
Lemon
Lemongrass
Peppermint
Spearmint
Tangerine

☑ Stress:

Basil
Bergamot
Frankincense
Ginger
Grapefruit
Lavender
Lemon
Roman Chamomile
Sandalwood

☑ Muscular:

Clove
Copaiba
Helichrysum
Idaho Balsam Fir
Lavender
Lemon
Peppermint
Vetiver
Wintergreen

☑ Muscles and Bones:

Basil
Cypress
Lavender
Lemongrass
Marjoram
Peppermint

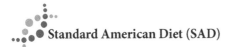 **Standard American Diet (SAD)**

The Standard American Diet (SAD) is very acidic, toxic laden, and causing a serious health crisis of obesity, diabetes, heart disease, and cancer. The continued consumption of acidic foods (sugar, meat, breads, caffeine, dairy, and alcohol) will eat away at our tissues and break down the essential functions, creating disease. Consuming a cleansing, alkaline diet is best for long term health goals.

So what is pH, and acid and alkaline? pH stands for potential hydrogen and it ranges from 0-14 with 7 being neutral. Below 7 is acidic, and above 7 is alkaline. The optimal blood level is 7.365 which is slightly alkaline. The pH level of our internal fluids influences every cell and decides our overall health. Much like farmers caring for and balancing the pH of their soil to grow clean food, the human body operates the same way. Acidic soil, much like an acidic body, grows weak plants and weak plants invite all kinds of pests that eat away at the plants. In the human body, an acidic environment invites illness and disease while an alkaline environment allows the systems of the body to function as best as possible. Disease cannot live in an alkaline environment therefore a nutritional base of alkaline foods is important to maintain optimal health. For athletes, maintaining a slightly alkaline body will help increase oxygen at a cellular level and ultimately lead to maximized performance. On the other hand, an acidic body acts in the complete opposite way, leading to a decrease of oxygen and causing you to deliver a sub-par performance.

"Take care of your body. It's the only place you have to live."
                    ~ **Jim Rohn**

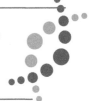

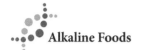 **Alkaline Foods**

Alkaline foods that are good for you are dark green, leafy vegetables, salads, fresh vegetables, nuts, seeds, low-sugar fruits and healthy oils such as olive oil. Alkaline foods produce better over-all health and a lean trim body. Acidic foods are those that are highly processed and refined foods, dairy, sugar-laden treats, caffeine, condiments, the whites (bread, rice, sugar, pasta), and fast foods. Aim for an 80-20 ratio (80% alkaline and 20% acidic foods) when choosing what you eat daily.

Categories of Alkalizing Foods

☑ **Allium** – garlic is anti-fungal, anti-bacterial and boosts immunity

☑ **Avocado** – essential fatty acids, amino acids and vitamins

☑ **Citrus** – lemon just squeezed in water to start the morning drink either hot or cold

☑ **Cruciferous vegetables** – brussels sprouts, cabbage, broccoli, cauliflower

☑ **Cucumber and celery** – in juices or smoothies to aid digestion and neutralize acid

☑ **Dark Green Leafy** – kale, spinach, Swiss chard, turnip greens, lettuces

☑ **Root vegetables** – carrots, beets, turnips, radishes, horseradish, rutabaga

Alkaline Foods

Avocado
Barley Grass
Broccoli
Cabbage
Capsicum/Bell Pepper/Pepper
Carrots
Cauliflower
Chlorella
Collard Greens
Dulce
Edible Flowers
Garlic

Horseradish
Kohlrabi
Lemons
Lettuce
Mustard Greens
Radishes
Rutabaga
Sprouts
Tomatoes
Wheat grass
Wild Greens

Alkaline Minerals

Calcium
Avocado
Broccoli
Celery
Kale
Mustard Greens
Spinach

Magnesium
Almonds
Basil
Cacao
Dill
Flax Seeds
Okra

Iron
Broccoli
Kale
Pumpkin Seeds
Quinoa
Spinach

Potassium
Avocado
Brussels Sprouts
Coconut Water
Figs
Kiwi
Tomatoes

Manganese
Chard
Cinnamon
Collard Greens
Garlic
Turmeric
Thyme

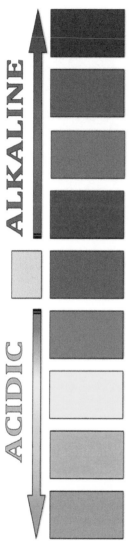

ACIDIC   ALKALINE

0 1 2 3 4 5 6 7.36 8 9 10 11 12 13 14

Healthy Body pH Range

Most Acid	Acid	Lowest Acid	Food Category	Lowest Alkaline	Alkaline	Most Alkaline
Aspartame Equal Nutra Sweet Sweet 'N Low	Brown Sugar White Sugar	Molasses Processed Honey	Sweeteners	Raw Honey Raw Sugar	Maple Syrup Rice Syrup	Stevia
Blueberries Cranberries Prunes	Sour Cherries Rhubarb	Plums Processed Fruit Juices	Fruits	Avocados Bananas Cherries Oranges Peaches Pineapples	Apples Berries Dates Figs Grapes Kiwi Melons Papaya Pears Raisins	Grapefruit Lemons Limes Mangoes Papayas Watermelons

Asparagus Broccoli Collard Garlic Onions Parsley Raw Spinach Seaweed Vegetable Juices	Beets Carob Celery Green Beans Lettuce Okra Squash Sweet Potato Zucchini	Cabbage Carrots Fresh Corn Mushrooms Olives Peas Potato Skins Tomatoes	**Beans Legumes Vegetables**	Cooked Spinach Kidney Beans String Beans	Lima Beans Navy Beans Pinto Beans Potatoes (without skins)	Chocolate
	Almonds	Chestnuts	**Nuts Seeds**	Pumpkin Seeds Sunflower Seeds	Cashews Pecans	Peanuts Walnuts
Olive Oil	Flax Seed Oil		**Oils**	Corn Oil		
		Amaranth Millet Quinoa Wild Rice	**Cereals Grains**	Bread Brown Rice Spelt Sprouted Wheat	Buckwheat Corn Oats Rye White Rice	Pasta Pastries Wheat White Flour
			Meats	Cold Water Fish Salmon Tuna Venison	Chicken Lamb Turkey	Beef Pork Shellfish
	Breast Milk	Goat Cheese Goat Milk Soy Milk Whey	**Eggs Dairy**	Butter Buttermilk Cottage Cheese Eggs Yogurt	Raw Milk	Cheese Homogenized Milk Ice Cream
Herb Teas Lemon Water	Green Tea	Ginger Tea	**Beverages**	Almond Milk Coconut Milk Rice Milk Tea	Coffee	Wine

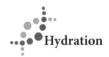

Hydration

Hydration is an incredibly huge part of our means to survival and who we are. Try living without water for a couple days. From a performance standpoint, hydration can be regarded as the main variable that can make or break the ultimate result and is extremely important in the regeneration process. The human body is made up of about 70% water. When dehydrated, that number can easily drop to 50-60%. Dehydration can slow down your metabolism, elevate stress hormones, and intensify inflammation and muscle soreness. A properly hydrated body ensures your blood is the proper consistency. When the cells are well hydrated, the cells will remain in an alkaline state, which is preferred.

Here are a few facts regarding hydration

- 75% of Americans are chronically dehydrated
- A single glass of water will eliminate midnight munchies for almost 100% of dieters that were studied in a University of Washington study
- Feeling thirsty is frequently mistaken for hunger
- A lack of water intake is the #1 cause of daytime fatigue
- A mere 2% decrease in body water can aggravate short-term memory, decrease basic math skills, and cause difficulty concentrating on the computer screen or printed paper
- Slight dehydration can slow down your metabolism
- Drinking the recommended amount of water daily can decrease the risk of colon cancer, breast cancer, and bladder cancer

Rehydrating your body is very important as well as replacing the proper minerals. Hyponatremia, a reduction in the salt level in the blood, is an electrolyte imbalance causing vomiting, headache, muscle weakness, lethargy, and cramps. In more serious situations, seizures or coma may occur. Depending on how many raw fruits and vegetables you are consuming religiously, you might not have to drink as much fluid as you think, as the raw whole foods are naturally filled with water and an abundance of minerals. These are considered to be hydrating foods. On the other hand, a diet that consists of foods cooked at high temperatures, processed grains and dry foods actually removes moisture from the cells and therefore would require drinking more water. They would be considered dehydrating foods.

As an athlete, you sweat out nutrients, called electrolytes, along with water when you train hard. Electrolytes are the essential nutrients that affect the amount of water in your body, the acidity (or pH level) of your blood, and your muscle function.

To maximize your body's efficiency, follow this rule of thumb for water consumption

- ☑ Drink 2 glasses after awakening to initiate the internal organs. Adding sliced lemon or therapeutic grade essential oil of lemon will aid in the detoxification process.
- ☑ Drink 1 glass approximately 30 minutes before a meal to aid with digestion.
- ☑ Drink 1 glass before taking a relaxing bath (preferably in Epsom salts and therapeutic grade essential oils) to help lower blood pressure.
- ☑ Drink 1 glass before retiring for the night to avoid heart related issues.

Without getting too deep into the different types of water, it is extremely important to try and find the cleanest water available. Whether it's spring water, filtered water, reverse osmosis or distilled, be sure it is truly pure clean water. Distilled water is the most controversial, yet is the closest one to actually being pure H2O as it contains no minerals or no toxic chemicals. Having your water tested for a variety of chemicals from fluoride and chlorine to lead is necessary. Consider a water purifier/filtration system attached to the faucet or purchase an external system.

Of course, with vigorous exercise from a morning skate to a full out game, you should definitely maintain a good water intake. The hydration process is something that must be constantly monitored for optimum results in competition. This process begins much sooner than the start of the game or competition as the proper foundation must be laid to be properly prepared. Throughout all practices or games you must continue to listen to your body whether it needs to be topped off with water or natural sugars and electrolytes. Once your body becomes dehydrated it's usually too late as performance drops and your body begins to cramp up. Don't let dehydration be the difference between winning or losing a game or winning or losing a championship.

Hydrating foods consist of

Cucumber	96%	water
Watermelon	96%	"
Pineapple	95%	"
Lettuce	95%	"
Blueberries	95%	"
Celery	95%	"
Tomatoes	94%	"
Pear	92%	"
Grapefruit	90%	"
Melon	89%	"

But what about **sport drinks** that you see advertised as the drink to keep you hydrated and balanced?

Typically **sports drinks** contain High Fructose Corn Syrup (HFCS), sodium, artificial colors and flavors. Sports drinks are 30 times more erosive to teeth than water. The citric acid will soften tooth enamel which brushing can then damage further.

A homemade **Healthy Electrolyte Drink** is tasty and will replenish sodium, potassium, magnesium and calcium. (see Hydration Recipes). These drinks are very easy to make without any negative side effects.

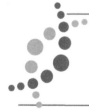

"Water is the most neglected nutrient in your diet but one of the most vital."
~ **Kelly Barton**

Coconut water contains natural electrolytes, enzymes, trace elements, amino acids and antioxidants. It is anti-inflammatory and has properties to help lower blood pressure. Because coconut water is high in sugar, limit intake to after a long duration of cardio.

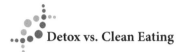 Detox vs. Clean Eating

Detox is the process, real or perceived, of removing toxins from the body (Wikipedia). Toxins are substances produced by living cells or organisms capable of causing disease when introduced into the body tissues. Toxins are a growing concern in the 21st century. We acquire them from the environment through the air we breathe, water we drink, household cleaning products and chemicals from air-tight housing, medications (over-the-counter and prescribed), radiation, and processed foods. **Detox**ification is typically recommended at least once a year if not with each season. Winter is usually not a good time since your body works on rebuilding and not cleansing. For athletes this would be something that should not be done during the season but rather at the end of it before you hit the ground running back into training mode. Popular magazines, top selling books, and online **detox**ification programs can help with the body's natural cleansing process by changing consumption habits.

So when do you need to **detox**? It is recommended for symptoms including but not limited to

1. Fatigue
2. Skin irritation (eczema, dermatitis)
3. Intestinal issues (constipation, bloating)
4. Hormonal issues
5. Allergies
6. Dark circles under the eyes, puffiness
7. Low-grade infections
8. Brain fog or mental confusion

No one **detox** program can work for everyone. Every body is unique. Some of the **detox** programs available are

1. Juice cleanse
2. Master cleanse
3. Hypoallergenic detox
4. Smoothie cleanse
5. Sugar detox
6. Fasting

There are certain foods that are naturally incorporated into some **detox** programs that help to cleanse the body. These foods, as you will see, are a part of **eating clean** as well.

1.	Artichokes	9.	Red bell pepper
2.	Broccoli	10.	Sunflower seeds
3.	Citrus fruit	11.	Turmeric
4.	Cucumber	12.	Turnip greens
5.	Garlic	13.	Walnuts
6.	Grapefruit	14.	Watercress
7.	Lentils	15.	Whole grains
8.	Mung beans		

With any **detox**ification program, hydration is crucial. (see Hydration Recipes for Detox Waters)

These programs can last from 2-3 days, 3-5 days, 1 week, or longer. You may not feel well during the **detox** process caused by intestinal issues, increased fatigue, and headaches. This is a natural process as your body is eliminating foreign toxins that have been present inside your body for a long time. Before starting any **detox** program, consult your health care practitioner if you have any questions or to decide if it is right for you. Discretion should be taken regarding any **detox** program in those with chronic degenerative conditions, cancer, arthritis, diabetes, chronic fatigue, or tuberculosis, during pregnancy or with nursing mothers, and children. Upon completing a **detox** program, it is recommended to gradually return to "normal" eating.

But what is considered "normal" eating? Going back to the old, not-so-healthy foods you ate before the **detox** program you just completed will only lead you back down the road to the above mentioned symptoms. Depending on the **detox** program, I am sure you do not want to end up there again.

By **eating clean** you keep your body in a constant state of detoxification and healing. It's a better way to allow your body to heal naturally. Again, every body is unique. We encourage athletes to nourish your body from the inside out with healthy whole foods and fluids while eliminating triggers that cause stress on the kidneys, liver, lungs, intestines, lymph and skin. It's suggested for life long health and wellness, creating balance in your body which **eating clean** promotes. "Where there's food, there's life."

So what do we mean by **eating clean**?

Eating clean is a lifestyle. Eating clean depends on a few simple concepts including

1. Eating plenty of fresh vegetables (6-10 servings) and fruits (2-3 servings) for fiber, vitamins, nutrients and enzymes.
2. Eating healthy fats every day such as avocado and wild caught salmon.
3. Eating a combination of lean protein and complete carbohydrates at each meal.
4. Strict following of proper portion sizes.
5. Eating breakfast daily, within an hour of rising.
6. Drinking pure water, approximately 2-3 liters or half your body weight in ounces.
7. Eating plenty of fiber.
8. Being prepared. Carry a small cooler packed with clean foods each day.
9. Stocking healthy food in the house – you can't eat poorly if it isn't there.
10. Prepping your meals in advance to avoid temptations.

"All disease begins in the gut."
~ **Hippocrates**

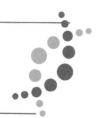

Eating clean also means eliminating

1. Processed foods, particularly those with white flour and sugar.
2. Chemically charged foods from pesticides and herbicides.
3. Foods containing preservatives and artificial sugars.
4. Soda and other sugary drinks like juices.
5. Excessive amounts of alcohol.
6. Saturated and trans-fats.
7. All calorie-dense foods containing little or no nutritional value.
8. Super-sizing your meals.
9. Products labeled "low-fat or "reduced fat."
10. Coffee and caffeine.

Eating clean is a process and is not something that happens overnight. Be open to change. Start slowly by adding more and more alkaline foods to your daily intake versus trying to do it all at once. By going more slowly, you will not feel like you are depriving yourself and you will start feeling stronger with each and every new day. The cramming technique seems to be an effective method for many people. It is simply cramming in more alkaline forming, plant based foods and cramming out acidic forming, highly processed and inflammatory foods. Listening to your body as to what works and what doesn't work takes time. Pick one new item to try weekly. **Eating clean** does everything a **detox** does but it continues day after day allowing your body to feel balanced. Other benefits of **eating clean** can include weight loss, fat loss, improved sleep, clearer skin, increased energy, better focus, shinier hair and, most importantly, overall health.

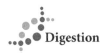 **Digestion**

The human body is incredibly designed when it is balanced and functioning at an optimum level. Eating is a means of energy and ultimately survival, however, the important key thing to understand is not all foods are digested and absorbed in the same manner. To fully understand how to maximize energy from food, we must take a quick glance at the digestive process.

Digestion is the breaking down of food, mechanically and chemically, in the gastrointestinal tract into portions small enough to be consumed (absorbed) by your body. Absorption is what moves those nutrients, including water and electrolytes, across the intestinal wall and into the blood and lymph. Digestion is a whole body system and does not act by itself. The digestive process starts in the mouth with chewing and saliva. Chew bites of food until it is mostly liquid. This may take anywhere from 20-30 chews or more. The food then moves through the gastrointestinal tract by means of a wave-like motion called peristalsis. This process is created through **balance** in the gut.

Creating **balance** in the gut will help relieve any digestive symptoms that you may have such as diarrhea, constipation, irritable bowel syndrome and other inflammatory bowel diseases. There is a four step process to help heal imbalances and are known as the **"4 R's."**

1. **Remove** foods, stress, toxins and bacteria causing digestive issues
2. **Replace** with healing, anti-inflammatory foods
3. **Repair** damage with specific supplements prescribed by your health care provider
4. **Rebalance** the gut with probiotics

In the quest to maximize general health and performance on all levels, incorporating more high quality organic whole foods is extremely important as these foods require less work to digest and ultimately output more energy. I call these **ENERGY +** foods. These foods are mainly alkaline forming in the body and limit digestive stress as the body doesn't waste much energy digesting them. On the other hand, refined sugars, processed foods and foods that are denatured because of high temperature cooking require more energy to digest and total output of energy is much lower. I call these **ENERGY** – foods. These foods are highly acidic forming in the body and increase digestive stress. All dead, processed and denatured foods have an acid impact on the body as well as contain toxins which lead to premature aging and cell degeneration. Wild and grass fed protein sources require more energy to digest so choose your portion of meat wisely. Six ounces of lean properly farmed meat is more than plenty for one meal as you don't want your body going into overdrive.

Digestive health consists of

1. Fiber – both whole and unprocessed
2. Hydration/water
3. Probiotics (through fermented vegetables - sauerkraut, kimchi, kombucha, apple cider vinegar, miso, or supplementation)
4. Eating slowly by taking small bites
5. Add spice to assist in the decrease of inflammation (black pepper, cardamom, coriander, cumin, turmeric)
6. Relaxation and meditation (music, walking, bathing, stress reduction, breath, self-massage, conversation)

Oxalic Acid

Some vegetables contain **oxalic acid** making the nutrients harder to digest and can possibly take out essential minerals such as calcium from the bones. It is possible that this acid can cause irritation to the digestive system, stomach and kidneys if eaten on a regular basis. The majority of people will not be affected by these foods. Those who do have a family history of osteoporosis, arthritis or mineral absorption issues may want to limit their consumption or alternate with lower oxalate vegetables. This will provide a variety of nutrients and will maximize overall calcium absorption.

Vegetables high in oxalic acid include
>Beet and beet greens
>Bell peppers
>Chives
>Parsley
>Rhubarb
>Spinach
>Swiss chard

Vegetables low in oxalic acid include
>Arugula
>Bok choy
>Kale
>Romaine
>Turnip greens

Other foods containing oxalic acid include
>Chocolate
>Cocoa
>Coffee
>Cranberries
>Peanuts
>Strawberries

Phytic Acid

Some grains, legumes and seeds contain **phytic acid** that can attach to minerals and proteins lessening the body's capability to absorb and efficiently use these nutrients (calcium, zinc, iron, magnesium and copper). To help offset **phytic acid** in grains and legumes, it is recommended to presoak for a minimum of one hour, drain, and add new water before cooking to allow for better digestibility of the complex carbohydrate. The longer grains soak, the more nutritious the grain becomes making it easier to digest. Another way to help counteract the acidity is to add a piece of Kombu (sea vegetable) or sea salt to the cooking process. Kombu increases the minerals, digestibility, tenderness, and decreases gas.

Smaller grains (quinoa, amaranth, teff and millet) are higher in protein and gluten-free. Brown, jasmine and wild rice are also gluten-free.

Legumes to presoak include
> Black beans
> Black-eyed peas
> Chickpeas (garbanzo beans)
> Great Northern beans
> Kidney beans
> Pinto beans
> Red beans
> Soy beans
> Split peas

Not All Calories Are Created Equal

Calories are needed to provide the body with energy for proper functioning.

Fat	1 gram = 9 calories ·
Protein	1 gram = 4 calories
Carbohydrates	1 gram = 4 calories

A combination of high quality fat, high fiber, low glycemic carbohydrates, and clean, lean protein from whole unprocessed foods over the course of the day will slow the digestive process so your energy will last longer throughout the day. Eating foods from all colors of the rainbow, involving the five tastes (sweet, sour, salty, bitter and umami), eating a variety of foods that are locally grown, seasonal consumption, and eating mindfully will create the balance necessary to produce the healthy body necessary for athletic competition.

Fat comes from seeds, nuts and some fruit including

Avocado
Coconut milk or oil
Olive oil, olives
Raw nuts
Raw seeds (hemp, chia, flax)
Wild cold water fish

Approximately 25-30% of calories should come from fat.

Types of fat

Saturated fat – mainly found in foods of animal source (red meat, poultry and dairy products); also found in some plant sources (coconut oil). Some are better for health than others and should be no more than 10% of calories.

Trans fat – found in processed foods (packaged and desserts), fried foods and shortening. Listed on packaging as "partially hydrogenated vegetable oil." Trans fats have been associated with elevated LDL ("bad" cholesterol levels) and lower HDL ("good" cholesterol levels).

Polyunsaturated fatty acids (PUFAs) – consists of omega -3 fatty acids (found in fatty fish, for example wild caught salmon, and plant based foods such as flaxseed and walnuts) and omega-6 fatty acids (found in vegetable oils like corn). PUFAs may help lower total cholesterol and decrease the risk of heart disease.

Monounsaturated fatty acids (MUFAs) – found in plant foods, for example avocados, olive oil and nuts. MUFAs may lower LDL levels and decrease the risk of heart disease.

Carbohydrates come from fruits, vegetables, legumes and grains.

Complex carbohydrates provide the major source of energy, accounting for 45-65% of calories daily. Complex carbohydrates consist of high fiber foods which aid in digestion, help to stabilize blood sugar levels, and keep you satisfied longer after your meal. Aim for 31.5 grams of fiber daily (beans, vegetables, fruit, whole grains). If you need to increase your fiber intake, increase by 5 grams weekly.

Simple carbohydrates are just that – simple. Made up of refined, processed flour and sugar for the most part, giving an instant boost of energy. Simple carbohydrates can lead to cravings and over eating, blood sugar swings affecting your mood, and weight gain.

High fiber, low glycemic carbohydrates

Adzuki beans
Apples
Beets
Berries
Black beans
Brown rice
Carrots
Chick peas
Hummus
Kidney beans
Lentils
Pumpkin
Quinoa
Squash
Sweet potato
Tomatoes

Protein comes from plants, fish, eggs and lean meats, poultry, and dairy.

Research shows that vegetarians and vegans get 70% more protein than needed daily.

Approximately 40 – 70 grams of protein daily (1/2 gram of protein per pound of lean body mass) should make up 25-30% of your daily calories. Some sources of clean, lean protein are chicken breast, grass-fed beef and pork, wild caught salmon and scallops.

A Calorie Is Not A Calorie

As you might assume the calories in an organic banana, which is an **ENERGY** + food, would not be equal to a chocolate bar which is **ENERGY** – food. So consciously choose foods that have whole nutrition as opposed to refined and processed foods. All dead, processed and denatured foods are empty foods with no usable nutrients however they still maintain caloric value. This would explain the obesity epidemic we see today, as the western diet consists mainly of processed and denatured foods.

Checking the number of calories on the ingredient label is a common occurrence when picking up a product in the grocery store. But where the calories come from is far more important than actually counting them. The number of calories needed will vary from person to person depending on how fast your metabolism is and how much you exercise daily. And it is unique to each and every one of us. Vigorous exercise (morning skate, strength training, and game) requires increased energy thus increased calories.

But again…a calorie is not a calorie. Let's look at snacks. Take a piece (approximately 4 ounces) of frosted chocolate cake. That is approximately 415 calories and it's loaded with sugar, white flour, and tons of simple carbohydrates. Now let's look at ½ cup broccoli (15 calories) dipped in 1 Tbsp. hummus (23 calories) for a total of 38 calories. This snack is nutrient rich with protein, healthy fat, fiber, and complex carbohydrates.

Calories need to be nutrient rich to provide the body with the essential means to keep us healthy and our immune system functioning properly.

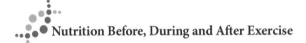

Nutrition Before, During and After Exercise

Whether you are a professional hockey player, a high school athlete, or a weekend warrior, what you eat before, during, and after exercise can make all the difference in how well your body, your temple, will perform and recover.

Nutrition Before Exercise

Fueling up for any practice, game or training regimen requires preparation. It begins the day or night before with meals consisting of nutrient rich foods and proper rest. The following day it's important to have your pre-workout or pre-game snack or meal approximately 2-4 hours prior to the event. The foods that you choose should be easy to digest. If you choose a heavy or overly spicy meal, you could run the risk of feeling upset and bloated. Also, if the meal isn't digested before or shortly into the event, your meal could be stuck in your stomach and not accessible to the muscles for much needed fuel. Any undigested food left in the stomach can sit there heavily creating fatigue and abdominal muscle spasms.

In general, you should aim for meals or snacks consisting of fat, fiber and protein as this combination will keep you feeling fuller longer. Pre-game though, you want a lower fat, fiber and protein content. Too much protein can lead to muscle cramping and decreased endurance. Protein is necessary for muscle building and not needed for fuel. A simple carbohydrate will be the healthiest choice such as a fruit which burns more slowly increasing effectiveness. Adding a fatty acid such as coconut oil will provide quick energy to burn as fuel in the liver. An example of a pre-game snack would be dates filled with coconut oil.

Nutrition Before, During And After

Proper hydration before, during and after game time will decrease the stress on the body allowing it to work harder, perform better, and recover quicker. (see Hydration and Hydration Recipes) Much needed electrolytes will decrease muscle cramping and spasms allowing for better performance. Pure water is important as are electrolytes that can be found in coconut water and homemade hydration drinks helping to maintain smooth muscle contractions and energy levels. What you consume for fuel and hydration is totally in your hands. No one is going to do it for you. So listening to your body is once again extremely important because it can be the difference between an elite performance or a very mediocre one. Fuel up wisely.

Nutrition After Exercise

After a hard morning skate or game, you want to eat a meal within 30 – 45 minutes for cellular reconstruction and recovery. Your meal should consist of high quality food, including 1 part protein to 4 parts carbohydrate. A whole food shake consisting of 1 piece of fruit, a large handful of your favorite greens and a handful of hemp seeds or raw almonds all blended up is a great way to refuel immediately following any physical exercise. Too much protein at this time will slow down recovery and should come from an alkaline source (see pH Chart).

An hour later, you still don't want to indulge in a large meal. Large amounts of food require an increase of blood to the stomach causing it to work harder while digesting. Oxygen is needed in the bloodstream so the muscles can recover. Post-game or post exercise nutrition needs alkalizing foods to repair the body by decreasing lactic acid buildup and physical stress. Another quick and easy snack would be to blend a frozen banana with 1 cup almond milk and 1 cup of kale.

"Food Is Fuel"

A **balance** of nutrients comes into play.

- ☑ Consider a lean protein for muscle repair (organic chicken, wild caught fish, nuts and seeds such as hemp)

- ☑ A whole grain to nourish muscle tissue (brown rice, millet, quinoa)

- ☑ Lots of produce to supply much needed whole foods (colorful vegetables, dark green leafy vegetables, apples)

- ☑ A healthy fat to aid in healing and circulation (avocado, wild caught fish, coconut oil, nuts, olive oil)

- ☑ More fluids for rehydration

Treat your body, your temple, to perform its best possible. Not only does this mean providing nutrient rich wholesome foods but it also means knowing what not to put into your body. Sugar creates inflammation in the body and can be found in numerous processed foods and drink. Sugars can lead to the production of fat specifically around the middle.

"Exercise is king. Nutrition is queen.
Put them together and you've got a kingdom."
~ **Jack LaLanne**

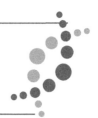

Travel

Preparation is a key component in achieving success no matter what job you currently hold. Athlete or not, we are constantly on the move and most of us tend to be on the road more often than not. When traveling, **eating clean** can definitely be a challenge. Preparation done the day before traveling to away games is a must. A trip to the grocery store, health food store or farmer's market, with list in hand, will promote healthy purchases leading to a body ready for energetic action on the ice. Meals in a jar or travel wraps (see Recipes) prepared in advance will provide the necessary nutrients. It's just a matter of preparing foods ahead of time. I recommend a small, hard cooler to bring along to any away event.

Other tools that you can bring along are a small blender to make smoothies. Whenever I travel for overnights, whether it is by car or plane, I always bring my blender with pre-packaged baggies of hemp protein, gogi berries, chia seeds, flax seeds, and cacao nibs. Add pure water and you're set. Also, a small knife and cutting board that fit in your cooler can be used for cutting veggies or fruit.

Snacks can also be packed for travel. Some options include

Almonds	*Grapefruit*
Apples	*Grapes*
Avocados with cottage cheese	*Greek yogurt with fresh berries*
Banana with nut butter	*Hemp seeds*
Bananas	*Peaches*
Berries	*Pecans*
Cashews	*Pistachios*
Clementine	*Pre-made salad*
Dark chocolate	*Trail Mix*
Fresh fruit smoothie	*Veggies and guacamole*
Gogi berries	*Veggies and homemade dressing*
Granola	*Veggies and hummus*

Additional travel options

Individual packets of oatmeal
Juices made from green powders – just add water
Foil packed wild salmon

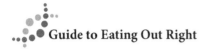

Options will vary depending on the restaurant, so do your best and choose wisely.

Appetizers

Appetizers are a great way to start out a leisurely meal, but can also derail your good intentions.

Don't Order

- ☒ Anything fried. Fried foods are a favorite but will do damage that even the most intense workout won't undo.
- ☒ Creamy dips. These are filled with fat and usually come with something fried to dip in it.
- ☒ Bread. It comes smothered in cheese or seeped in butter, and even when it's plain it fills you up with more carbohydrates than your body needs.

Do Order

- ☑ Green Salad. Ask for a very light dressing or simply olive oil and balsamic vinegar. No croutons.
- ☑ Antipasto. A plate of thinly sliced meats, olives and cheese will start you off with some protein.
- ☑ Lettuce wraps. These are delicious, protein filled and low in carbohydrates.

*"By failing to prepare,
you are preparing to fail."*

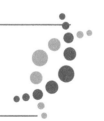

Beverages

Calories in drinks typically don't fill you up and you end up taking in far more calories than expected.

Don't Order

- ☒ Regular or diet soda. On one hand you are drinking corn syrup through a straw, on the other you're drinking chemicals that cause you to crave sweets.
- ☒ Sweetened tea. You may feel better ordering iced tea, but if it's sweetened you may as well be drinking fully loaded soda.

Do Order

- ☑ Water. Seriously!! Water is the best beverage of all!!
- ☑ Unsweetened iced tea. Don't ruin it by adding a packet of sugar. Enjoy the natural flavor and sweetness of the tea.

Entrees

Here is where real damage can occur. Carb-loaded meals leave you feeling heavy and lethargic. When eating better, you'll experience the light, energetic way it makes your body feel afterwards.

Don't Order

- ☒ Pasta. It doesn't matter if it comes with red or white sauce, meat or veggies.
- ☒ Pizza. Another dish that contains more carbohydrates than needed. If craving pizza toppings, then order those over a salad.
- ☒ Burgers. If you are craving a burger, then remove the bun and ditch the fries, and wrap your patty in lettuce.

Do Order

- ☑ Lean meat with vegetables. Fish, steak or chicken (you choose) and pair it with green vegetables.
- ☑ Salad with protein. Ask for a light dressing and make sure you have a nice protein source on top.
- ☑ Soup and salad. Stick with broth-based soups containing protein.

The most important thing to remember is to PREPARE ahead of time. This will keep you and your body on track.

Guide to Food Labels

Reading and understanding food labels can be intimidating. A number of the terms are strictly for marketing purposes, whereas others are approved by the Food and Drug Administration (FDA) regulating grocery items and nutritional information such as calories, vitamins and fat content, or the United States Department of Agriculture (USDA) who oversees meats, animal products, grains and produce. The simplest and most effective way to avoid any confusion with food labels would be to consume a strict diet of whole foods as fresh produce does not have food labels. However in today's world this is an unrealistic goal as consuming at least a few processed foods is inevitable.

Before looking at the nutritional profile of the food you are analyzing start by looking at the list of ingredients that's below it. If the list looks anything like the following paragraph you can't even pronounce, it should be an immediate red flag. It is littered with refined and denatured parts of food, chemicals, fillers and more garbage. In this example different types of sugar is listed multiple times under different names. It has absolutely no nutrition at all, just empty calories. Compare that ingredient list with this list of an organic spirulina energy bar and it surely doesn't take a rocket scientist to figure out which one is the cleaner, healthier and wiser choice. All the ingredients listed are nutrient rich organic whole foods. This label also mentions a few other important things for the conscious consumer such as No GMO, gluten free and dried under 105 degrees, which means this food still maintains most of its nutrition.

"Before looking at the nutritional profile of the food you are analyzing start by looking at the list of ingredients that's below."

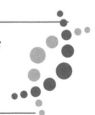

INGREDIENTS: ENRICHED FLOUR (WHEAT FLOUR, NIACIN, REDUCED IRON, THIAMIN MONONITRATE [VITAMIN B_1], RIBOFLAVIN [VITAMIN B_2], FOLIC ACID), CORN SYRUP, SUGAR, SOYBEAN AND PALM OIL (WITH TBHQ FOR FRESHNESS), CORN SYRUP SOLIDS, DEXTROSE, HIGH FRUCTOSE CORN SYRUP, FRUCTOSE, GLYCERIN, CONTAINS 2% OR LESS OF COCOA (PROCESSED WITH ALKALI), POLYDEXTROSE, MODIFIED CORN STARCH, SALT, DRIED CREAM, CALCIUM CARBONATE, CORNSTARCH, LEAVENING (BAKING SODA, SODIUM ACID PYROPHOSPHATE, MONOCALCIUM PHOSPHATE, CALCIUM SULFATE), DISTILLED MONOGLYCERIDES, HYDROGENATED PALM KERNEL OIL, SODIUM STEAROYL LACTYLATE, GELATIN, COLOR ADDED, SOY LECITHIN, DATEM, NATURAL AND ARTIFICIAL FLAVOR, VANILLA EXTRACT, CARNAUBA WAX, XANTHAN GUM, VITAMIN A PALMITATE, YELLOW #5 LAKE, RED #40 LAKE, CARAMEL COLOR, NIACINAMIDE, BLUE #2 LAKE, REDUCED IRON, YELLOW #6 LAKE, PYRIDOXINE HYDROCHLORIDE (VITAMIN B_6), RIBOFLAVIN (VITAMIN B_2), THIAMIN HYDROCHLORIDE (VITAMIN B_1), CITRIC ACID, FOLIC ACID, RED #40, YELLOW #5, YELLOW #6, BLUE #2, BLUE #1.

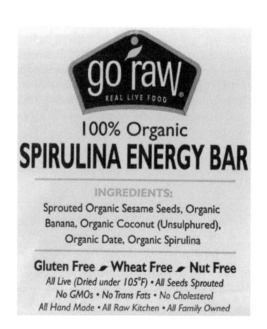

go raw

REAL LIVE FOOD

100% Organic

SPIRULINA ENERGY BAR

INGREDIENTS:

Sprouted Organic Sesame Seeds, Organic
Banana, Organic Coconut (Unsulphured),
Organic Date, Organic Spirulina

Gluten Free ✔ Wheat Free ✔ Nut Free

*All Live (Dried under 105°F) • All Seeds Sprouted
No GMOs • No Trans Fats • No Cholesterol
All Hand Made • All Raw Kitchen • All Family Owned*

Once you have evaluated the actual ingredients that make up your food, it is wise to take a look at the actual nutrition facts, which are usually before the list of ingredients. Most labels break down foods into simple macro nutrients like calories, fat, carbohydrate, protein and a few others like sugar which is an important one to understand. Start by acknowledging the amount of servings per container as many companies use this to mask the total amount of calories. While at first glance you might think it is a low calorie food, once you add up the amount of servings, it soon becomes a high calorie food. Sugar and sodium are usually the two ingredients that make most processed foods problematic so take a good look at how much the food contains. Do your best to choose high fiber and low calorie foods. Again using some common sense will surely help you in choosing foods wisely.

Nutrition Facts

Serving Size ½ cup (114g)
Servings Per Container 4

Amount Per Serving

Calories 90	Calories from Fat 30

	% Daily Value*
Total Fat 3g	5%
Saturated Fat 0g	0%
Cholesterol 0mg	0%
Sodium 300mg	13%
Total Carbohydrate 13g	4%
Dietary Fiber 3g	12%
Sugars 3g	
Protein 3g	

Vitamin A 80%	•	Vitamin C 60%	
Calcium 4%	•	Iron 4%	

*Percent Daily Values are based on a 2,000 calorie diet. Your daily values may be higher or lower depending on your caloric needs:

	Calories:	2,000	2,500
Total Fat	Less than	65g	80g
Sat Fat	Less than	20g	25g
Cholesterol	Less than	300mg	300mg
Sodium	Less than	2,400mg	2,400mg
Total Carbohydrate		300g	375g
Dietary Fiber		25g	30g

Calories per gram:
Fat 9 • Carbohydrate 4 • Protein 4

The following are many of the terms used on food labels

☑ **Cage Free** – An unregulated label. The egg-laying hens are not put in cages but it doesn't mean they were freely roaming or even outdoors. Mainly, they are warehoused and packed in overcrowded barns usually in unsanitary conditions. Beak cutting is another inhumane practice under this label. Does not regulate feed or antibiotics.

☑ **Free Range or Free Roaming** – The USDA requires five minutes of "open-air" access a day. These animals have the ability to go outdoors but it doesn't mean that they actually did. There is no requirement regarding grass, dirt or space.

☑ **CAFOs (Confined Animal Feeding Operations)** – Beef, pork, chicken, turkey, etc. raised in a factory farm.

☑ **Barn Roaming** – These animals were not caged but they also were not free to go outside.

☑ **Grass-Fed** – A USDA standard requiring typically cows, goats and sheep to be able to graze, being fed a diet of only grass and forage, no grains.

☑ **Vegetarian-Fed** – A questionable label where the animals were not given any animal by-product but their diet may have included grains.

☑ **Certified Humane** – Says nothing about what type of diet was provided. The animals were not kept in cages, tethers or crates allowing free movement but it does not suggest they had the ability to go outdoors or enough room to walk around. Prohibits animal by-products in feed, growth promoters and the use of non-therapeutic antibiotics. Allows beak cutting.

☑ **Natural** – The product may not be comprised of any artificial ingredients/flavors, synthetic substances or added color. This term has no FDA guidelines so products can be heavily processed. For example, animals raised with growth hormone and antibiotics, or the use of high fructose syrup (sometimes called corn sugar) which is a natural substance but if produced from raw corn this requires many processing measures.

☑ **Naturally Grown** – Foods produced on relatively small farms that follow USDA Certified Organic methods of growing and sell locally.

☑ **No Hormones Administered** – No hormones were given to the cattle. It is illegal throughout the nation to use hormones in pigs or poultry.

☑ **No Antibiotics Added** – No antibiotics were administered even in sickness while raising the animals.

☑ **Fresh** – Used differently for different products. The products can include "approved" coatings or waxes, post-harvested approved pesticides, rinsing or applying a chlorine or mild acid wash, or ionizing radiation.

☑ **Certified Organic** – The animal had the ability to go outdoors and to bedding but it is unsure for how long. In raising these animals no hormones or antibiotics were administered.

☑ **100% Organic** – Every ingredient in the product was raised, harvested and processed in an organic environment and certified by the USDA.

☑ **Organic** – These products are 95% organic. The remaining 5% cannot contain growth hormones. The animals involved must never have been given hormones, antibiotics, or GMO grasses.

☑ **Made With** – The food product could include other ingredients besides what the front label says.

☑ **Made With Organic Ingredients** – At least 70% of ingredients are organically produced. The remaining 30% could be non-organic.

☑ **Good Source Of/Contains/Provides** – The food product needs to verify that a minimum of 10% of the vitamin or nutrient of the USDA's recommended daily allowance is included.

☑ **High Source Of/Rich In/Excellent Source Of** – The food product must contain a minimum of 20% of the vitamin or nutrient recommended by the USDA's daily allowance.

☑ **Animal Welfare Approved** – Prohibits cages and the use of antibiotics. Requires access to outdoors but the amount and quality can vary.

As you can see, there are many labels and even more than are located here. To make certain you are purchasing the best quality of meat, fruits and vegetables that you can, it is suggested you shop at the farmer's market where you can speak with the farmer directly.

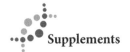 **Supplements**

Obviously, you want to eat as clean as possible and obtain a balanced, healthy lifestyle from a nutrient dense diet. Sometimes that doesn't always work out the way it's intended. You want your meals to contain high quality whole foods but occasionally you simply can't get all the nutrients you need from food. The quality of the soil where the plants were grown may be deficient in necessary minerals. There could be seasonal weather related issues from drought to heavy rains. Depending on the time it takes to get from the farm to your table, depending on where the foods are grown and harvested, you could lose valuable nutrients along the way.

So are supplements the answer? There is not a quick and easy response to that question. When you look at what a whole food can provide, you find a multitude of vitamins and minerals working **together** to provide you with the optimal nutritive value. When you look at a supplement, you are getting just that – the specific supplement as a **single** active ingredient. There typically are no other components associated with the supplement as there is in a whole food. So if you can, let nature do its job by eating whole nutrient dense foods to provide you with the quality and quantity your body needs.

There are numerous studies showing how some supplements may actually be beneficial for certain medical conditions or deficiencies as noted through blood work. Still you need to be cautious of study results as they could be no better than a pharmaceutical company looking to promote a medication.

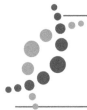 *"In recommending supplements, you want to look for a high quality product free of fillers, without contamination of heavy metals, and with appropriate dosing."*

In recommending supplements, you want to look for a high quality product free of fillers, without contamination of heavy metals, and with appropriate dosing. There are many brands and companies to choose from which makes this decision even more difficult. And then there is the cost. Supplements can be very expensive.

There are three supplements that may be needed

1. **Vitamin D3 (cholecalciferol)** – Vitamin D is essential for bone health, immunity and fat loss. Vitamin D3 is best synthesized by the human body from sunlight. It's important to have a blood test checking for Vitamin D 25-OH. This value can also be determined by where you live and if you use sunscreen. The reference range is 30 – 100 ng/ml. That is a very large range. What appears to be more acceptable is the range between 50 – 80 ng/ml.

2. **Omega 3 Fatty acids** – Omega-3's are helpful in reducing inflammation in the body. Foods associated with Omega-3's are fish (salmon, tuna, sardines) and certain nuts and seeds. Supplementation comes as fish oil capsules. As with fish, you need to look for wild-caught sources being wary of contamination from mercury and PCBs.

3. **Probiotic** – Probiotics are important in "gut" health as they support good bacteria. The bacteria in your gut can be thrown off by poor digestion, travel, diets high in sugar and artificial ingredients, environmental toxins, certain medications from antacids to pain medications, and the use of antibiotics. Natural probiotics consist of sauerkraut, kimchi, pickled ginger, organic miso, fermented vegetables and apple cider vinegar.

Body Balance in Review – Part Two

☑ The complexity of stress in today's everyday life plays havoc on your body affecting your hormones, affecting your sleep, affecting how you cope. Look to the many possibilities in the recovery from stress for improved balance.

☑ Nothing is better than a good night's sleep! Providing necessary energy, weight management, and a healthy immune system is key for recovery and performance.

☑ Mother Nature's gift of therapeutic grade essential oils is mankind's first medicine. Essential oils can aid in sleep, reduce inflammation, decrease anxiety, and bring balance.

☑ Consuming a cleansing, alkaline diet provides the necessary nutrients to achieve your health goals.

☑ Learn which foods and drinks are alkaline and acidic helping you to create balance in your food choices.

☑ Proper hydration with pure, clean water and hydrating foods will prevent muscle cramping, headache, and decrease inflammation.

☑ Each body is unique. Eating clean will nourish your body creating a natural detoxification one day at a time.

☑ Maximizing health and performance means looking at Energy + and Energy – foods. Digestive health improves with nutrient rich foods and is not determined by the number of calories consumed.

☑ The food that you eat before, during and after exercise can make all the difference in the world as to how you feel, how you recover and how you will be prepared for your next workout. Balancing your nutrients will determine the outcome of performance.

☑ Prepare! Prepare! Prepare!! Whether you're away for an overnight, a few days, or a week… preparation is vital and will keep your body on track.

☑ Reading labels can be daunting. My favorite label is one that consists of one item making the choice easy but in reality there are labels needing to be read and choices to be made.

☑ A whole food nutrient dense diet provides necessary vitamins and minerals. Supplements may be of benefit with occurring deficiencies.

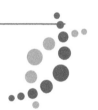

"Not-so-good choices and the fast pace of life create inflammatory triggers placing stress on major organs of the body."

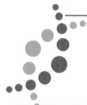

"Digestive health improves with nutrient rich foods and is not determined by the number of calories consumed."

Part Three

Imbalanced Body

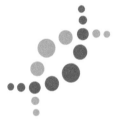

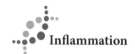 **Inflammation**

Living in today's high paced world can cause your body and mind to sometimes feel like life is occurring at an even faster pace than you would like. With that fast pace, it's too easy to stop to grab a quick bite to eat but it's not always the best choice. The quick choices that are out there, for the most part, consist of sugar, caffeine, refined flours, dairy, chemical food additives, environmental pollutants and pesticides. These not-so-good choices and the fast pace of life create inflammatory triggers placing stress on major organs of the body. Toxins build up stressing the kidneys, liver, colon, and lymphatic system. So what can you do to reduce the inflammation that is aging you?

First, it's important to understand what inflammation actually is and how you can take care of yourself to prevent inflammation from taking over your body faster than you would like.

There are two types of inflammation

1. The first is **acute** inflammation – the kind everyone knows. This type of inflammation occurs as a local reaction to illness or injury characterized by swelling, warmth, pain, loss of function, and redness. These characteristics are a part of your body's natural immune system protecting your body so that it will heal. Inflammation protects and heals by fighting infection, repairing damaged tissue, battling against damaging organisms, and protecting against toxins. In hockey, you're getting checked into the boards, dragged down to the ice, and are physically stressing your body simply from playing the game. Acute inflammation that does not resolve itself within a few days may mean that you are experiencing a more chronic type of inflammatory process on the body.

2. The second is **chronic** inflammation – the kind that appears to be linked to chronic disease such as heart disease, obesity, cancer, depression, autism, arthritis, gout, and dementia. Research has shown that inflammation plays a role in the growth of tumors, the advancement of hardening of the arteries, and insulin resistance.

There is a correlation between nutrition, lifestyle and inflammation. Reversing chronic health problems can occur by eating the proper foods, avoiding toxins, incorporating proper daily nutrients and adding beneficial physical movement. For athletes, battling inflammation daily is an ongoing thing. As an empowered athlete, it is your duty to stay on top of any acute inflammation you might have which requires constant maintenance. While applying ice on an acute injury may help temporarily, you need to remove inflammation from the inside out. This means a clean, nutrient dense diet consisting of anti-inflammatory foods and eliminating the inflammatory foods which are working against your body's natural ability to heal.

Top Anti-Inflammatory Foods

Celery: High in luteolin, a flavonoid, assists with inflammation in the brain.

Kale, Swiss Chard, Collards: High in anti-oxidants and Vitamin K. Add to smoothies for an extra dose of anti-inflammatory goodness.

Extra Virgin Olive Oil: High in oleocanthal, an anti-inflammatory compound, and heart-healthy monounsaturated fat. The best source is from the first pressing of the olives so aim to purchase the best possible.

Lentils: High in folate, a B vitamin that can assist in the reduction of homocysteine that has been connected with inflammation and heart disease.

Hemp Seeds: High in omega-3 fats and gamma-linolenic acid (GLA) which may increase the production of anti-inflammatory compounds. (see Hemp)

Grapefruit: High in flavonoids to help lower inflammation.

Tumeric: Curcumin, which gives turmeric (traditionally an Indian spice) its yellow color is an antioxidant and a known anti-inflammatory. It's easy to add a dash or two to curries soups, and stir-fries.

Ginger: A warming herb and spice helping with digestion and decreasing inflammation in the colon. Also aids in the reduction of swelling and pain in joints. Add a slice or two to smoothies for added zing.

Pistachios: High in vitamin B6 which decreases the level of CRP (C-Reactive Protein – an inflammatory marker) and oxidative injury, and high in monosaturated fatty acids.

Whole Grains: Brown rice, quinoa and buckwheat, for example, lower the level of CRP.

Beets: Multicolored assortment (red, orange, pink and yellow) provides Vitamin C, is heart healthy, protects against cancer and assists in reducing swelling.

Avocado: A healthy monounsaturated fat to reduce inflammation. Add to smoothies, salads, dressings, healthful puddings for additional creaminess.

Fatty fish: Fresh, wild-caught seafood such as salmon and mackerel either baked or broiled also are anti-inflammatory foods that add protein to your diet.

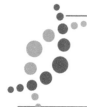

"Foods should be GMO-free, fresh, organic or locally grown."

More Anti-Inflammatory Foods

Almonds/almond butter
Apples
Asparagus
Avocados/avocado oil
Bee Pollen
Beets-red
Bell Peppers
Blueberries
Bok Choy
Broccoli
Brussels sprouts
Cabbage
Cantaloupe
Cauliflower
Cayenne
Chard
Cherries
Chicken
Chives
Cilantro
Cinnamon
Cloves
Cocoa
Coconut oil
Cod-wild caught
Collards
Cranberries
Cucumber
Cumin seeds
Extra virgin olive oil
Fennel bulb
Figs
Flaxseed (ground/oil)

Garlic
Ginger
Grapes
Green beans
Guava
Hazelnuts
Hemp seeds
Herring
Horseradish
Jicama
Kale
Kelp
Kiwi
Kumquats
Leeks
Legumes
Lemons
Lentils
Limes
Macadamia
Mackerel
Mint
Mulberries
Mushrooms
Olives
Onions
Oregano
Oysters
Papaya
Parsley
Peaches
Peas (fresh)
Pepper, black

Pineapple
Plums
Pumpkin
Quinoa
Radish
Raspberries
Rosemary
Rutabaga
Salmon-wild caught
Sardines
Seaweed
Sesame seeds
Sprouted seeds
Squash
Strawberries
Sweet potatoes
Thyme
Tomatoes
Tuna
Walnuts
Watermelon
Yam

Foods should be GMO-free, fresh, organic or locally grown.

Meats should be organic and not factory farmed.

Muscular Aches and Pains

A homemade anti-inflammatory/anti-oxidant paste that not only aids in muscular aches and pain but also helps to prevent heart disease (decrease cholesterol), and neurological diseases (such as Alzheimer's, Parkinson's and Multiple Sclerosis) is as follows

Ingredients:

⅓ cup honey (unpasteurized)
1 tsp. vanilla extract
2 ½ - 3 tsp. turmeric
1 tsp. cinnamon

Directions:

Mix all together until a paste is formed. Keep in a sealed container. Apply to affected area as needed.

Flotation Therapy

Flotation Therapy, with its unique therapeutic approach, was created over 50 years ago. This modality can decrease inflammation in joints, muscles and tissue pain, relaxes your muscles, decreases stress hormones (cortisol and adrenaline), increases relaxation and calmness, improves sleep and will improve recovery time and performance in an athlete.

A flotation therapy session usually lasts for 60 – 90 minutes with some staying for 2 – 3 hours. You basically stay until you are ready to get out. You start by lying back in a private pool with 10 inches of clean filtered water diffused with a Dead Sea Epsom salt blend. With this special blend, you are able to float with ease (promoting a feeling of weightlessness) while feeling totally relaxed. Flotation therapy is popular in Europe but is gaining attention here in the states.

Insomnia

Insomnia is the inability to fall asleep or sleep interrupted early. Even one night of not being able to fall asleep can throw off your hormones by increasing the stress hormone cortisol, and throwing off the fat-burning hormones as well.

It's very hard to turn off your mind and fall asleep on game night. For athletes, getting to sleep after a big game is often a struggle. Not returning home until 10:30 pm or later after a grueling effort can be hard on the body and the mind. The adrenaline is still flowing and your mind is racing reflecting on that game and looking onto the next. And if it's an away game, you might find yourself on the bus or plane, in a more than uncomfortable position. Sadly, there is no one answer to remedy this problem. Finding that balance for restful sleep is individual and can comprise of many actions.

Going to sleep on a full stomach is not recommended but there are some foods that can help with sleep on those difficult nights.

- ☑ Almonds contain magnesium that works as a natural muscle relaxant and de-stressor.
- ☑ Bananas are also rich in magnesium plus potassium and tryptophan (turkey on Thanksgiving which makes you drowsy on Thanksgiving) aids in sleep.
- ☑ Oatmeal is another magnesium and potassium rich food that tends to warm the soul creating calmness.
- ☑ Cherries and cherry products such as tart cherry juice have been found to increase melatonin improving sleep.
- ☑ Pumpkin seeds, another food high in magnesium, with a small apple can also aid in sleep.

Essential oils such as lavender and chamomile are very well known to help relax the body and promote sleep. (see Essential Oils page for more information.)

Caffeine

Caffeine is another controversial issue when it comes to diet and nutrition. It is a very powerful substance that can offer an energetic and stimulating feeling. Much like most things available for consumption, caffeine is often abused, leading to many different side effects. Caffeine, from coffee and other products, creates an acidic environment in the body (see pH Chart) playing havoc on the body's minerals. When consuming caffeinated beverages throughout the day, you end up basically flushing the balancing minerals out of your body. This also places stress on your immune system creating a "fight or flight" response from the production of adrenaline. When you run out of adrenaline, you may feel fatigued, anxious and irritable. This leads to consuming more caffeine and creates a vicious cycle. This up and down feeling can lead to adrenal fatigue and possibly adrenal burnout. Symptoms of adrenal issues include fatigue, depression, low blood sugar, muscle and joint pain, allergies, and chronic infections.

Brewed coffee contains a fair amount of caffeine and is considered highly acidic. The coffee bean contains oils that when roasted, can spoil. This in turn will cause the liver to be sluggish delaying the release of toxins from the body.

Caffeine is a stimulant that can also affect your sleep. It is recommended that you don't consume caffeine later than noon in order to have a restful night. But some athletes like the stimulant effect prior to a game as it can improve the central nervous system (CNS) output. Then, after arriving home from the rink on game night at 10:00 - 11:00 at night, sleep may be difficult to achieve. Not only are you still pumped up from the game but you might also be having the remaining effects of the caffeine. If you plan on using caffeine as an athlete, it is extremely important to listen to your body and know how much your body can tolerate to maintain maximum performance without compromising your mental state with anxiety and jitters. Some people are extremely sensitive to caffeine and consuming caffeine would clearly have a negative effect on everything from mood to mental state to performance.

Caffeine Pros and Cons

Pros
- ☑ Can enhance aerobic endurance
- ☑ May prevent motor deficits and brain degeneration, enhance brain function, and improve memory
- ☑ Protect against Parkinson's disease
- ☑ Decrease the risk of Type 2 Diabetes
- ☑ Decreases the cognitive decline linked with aging including the incidence of Alzheimer's disease when consumed moderately
- ☑ Improves the feeling of happiness, alertness, sociability, energy and a sense of overall well-being
- ☑ Provides antioxidants (1,299 mg. per 1-½ cups of daily coffee) protecting cells from damage

Cons
- ☒ Wrinkles skin prematurely due to dehydration
- ☒ Can lead to higher incidence of osteoporosis, due to the excretion of calcium in urine (approximately 5 mg. calcium lost from 6 oz. coffee). If drinking coffee, add 2 Tbsp. non-dairy milk (almond, hemp, or coconut) to counter balance these effects.
- ☒ Increases exposure to chemicals, pesticides and herbicides as coffee plants are heavily sprayed
- ☒ Can trigger migraine headaches
- ☒ Increases nervousness
- ☒ May cause or exacerbate sleep issues

"Caffeine is a stimulant that can also affect your sleep. It is recommended that you don't consume caffeine later than noon in order to have a restful night."

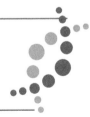

Caffeine

Coffee	8 oz. brewed	108 mg
Yerba Mate Tea	8 oz.	85 mg
Red Bull	8.46 oz.	80 mg
Monster Energy	8 oz.	80 mg
Espresso	1.5 oz. shot	77 mg
Instant Coffee	8 oz.	65-90 mg
Mountain Dew	12 oz.	54 mg
Black Tea	8 oz.	42 mg
Coca-Cola Classic	12 oz.	34 mg
White Tea	8 oz.	28 mg
Green Tea	8 oz.	25 mg
Kombucha Tea	8 oz.	24 mg
Dark Chocolate	1 oz.	20 mg
Decaffeinated Coffee	8 oz.	6 mg
Milk Chocolate	1 oz.	6 mg
Chocolate Milk	8 oz.	4 mg
Decaffeinated Green Tea	8 oz.	3 mg
White Chocolate	1 oz.	0 mg
Herbal Tea	8 oz.	0 mg

Caffeine Consumption Reduction

In reducing the amount of caffeine consumed on a daily basis, try these strategies:

- ☑ Drink green or white tea which has small amounts of caffeine

- ☑ Drink homemade green juices or smoothies before any caffeinated beverage as this will decrease the amount of caffeine needed for increased energy. By including green drinks consisting of kale, broccoli or spinach, you will be detoxifying the body naturally and providing a clean source of energy.

- ☑ Add raw cacao (fruit of the cacao tree) to smoothies or make a drink directly from this raw chocolate. Cacao has less caffeine, is energy boosting, contains magnesium (aids in normal bone health and a healthy immune system), copper, manganese, sulfur, essential fatty acids, antioxidant flavonoids, and has been considered by some as a superfood.

☑ Drink alternative herbal beverages such as Teeccino (an herbal coffee made from certified organic carob pods, barley and chicory, dates and figs, almonds, ramon seeds and dandelion root) or Postum (a roasted grain beverage, caffeine-free made from wheat bran, wheat, molasses and maltodextrin).

☑ If you must have your coffee, choose organic and try to cut back to one cup a day.

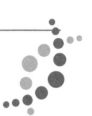

"Some people are extremely sensitive to caffeine and consuming caffeine would clearly have a negative effect on everything from mood to mental state to performance."

Dairy

Dairy seems to be one of the most controversial pieces of diet and nutrition. We all drank milk when we grew up because we were told it would help build strong bones. Dairy has been the go-to food for meeting all of our calcium needs. But the fact is, there are a variety of other food sources that are healthier and have fewer allergen possibilities and less gastrointestinal discomfort such as gas and bloating. Lactose intolerance currently affects approximately 75% of adults and appears to be on the rise. Dairy is also an acidic food. It's high in saturated fat, highly inflammatory, mucus forming and contains added synthetic growth hormones. Consuming dairy products can lead to many chronic diseases (such as Crohn's disease), coronary artery disease, asthma and allergies, eczema and acne, kidney stones, and may also activate malignant cell growth.

Let's put this into perspective. Cow's milk is for calves, not humans. For human babies, we have breast milk. Humans are the only species on earth that drink another mammal's milk and the only species that drinks milk after it has completed breast feeding. Cow's milk has three times the protein as breast milk so one may think that would be a good thing. Right? Not so much. Calves need cow's milk to grow into a 1200-1500 pound cow. Human babies thankfully don't grow to that extent. Thus, breast milk contains the perfect ingredients to grow happy and healthy children. As calves grow into cows, they don't continue to consume cow's milk. So why do humans have the need to consume milk? Casein, which is a protein in cow's milk, can generate and promote the growth of cancer cells as described by Dr. T. Colin Campbell.

All dairy products are incredibly well marketed. We have all seen the high profile celebrity with a milk mustache quoting milk does a body good. This couldn't be further from the truth. We have been misled and programmed to think that. Not only does drinking one of the fatter species on earth's milk seem a bit silly, if you have ever seen how animals today are factory farmed there is no way you could ever support it. These cattle are raised and slaughtered at CAFOs (concentrated animal feeding operation) with virtually no exercise, fed a diet of GMO corn and other grain when cows were meant to eat grass, and on top of that are pumped with steroids, growth hormones and antibiotics. Not exactly what you would qualify as clean eating.

Properly raised, grass fed cattle is clearly a much better alternative than conventionally farmed cattle however it remains a highly inflammatory food, and acidic and creates mucus in the body.

Calcium has also been touted as the answer to bone health. But in countries where there is a high intake of calcium specifically from dairy products, you will also find a higher incidence of osteoporosis. In order to maintain bone health, proper nutrition and physical activity are necessary and determine the calcium your body needs. Vitamin D is required for the absorption of calcium in the body. In an attempt to achieve the needed Vitamin D level, you must get out in the sunshine for approximately 20 minutes at least three times per week. Those who live in the northern atmospheres may find this difficult to obtain. A Vitamin D blood test will help determine if supplementation is needed.

Non-Dairy Milk Alternatives can be found in almost any store from the refrigerated dairy section to cartons on the shelf in the health food section. These milk alternatives come in all forms, from coconut milk to hemp milk to almond milk and many more. These can replace cow's milk especially if you have issues with lactose or are looking for a healthier substitute. There is an ingredient in the non-dairy milks that you should be aware of though. It is "carrageenan" which is used as a thickening agent and has stabilizing properties. Intestinal issues can occur in response to this addition. If you notice that your gut does not feel well after the intake of any of the non-dairy milks with this additive, it is highly recommended to discontinue. Non-dairy milks are very easy to make (see Recipes) and you can be guaranteed of its purity. Plus they taste wonderful!

"Non-dairy milk alternatives can replace cow's milk especially if you have issues with lactose or are looking for a healthier substitute."

Calcium Rich Foods

Almonds
Asparagus
Avocado
Black eyes peas
Blackstrap
  molasses
Bok choy
Brazil nuts
Broccoli
Brussels sprouts
Butternut squash
Cabbage
Celery

Chia seeds
Coconut meat
Collard greens
Dates
Figs
Kale
Kiwi
Kohlrabi
Kumquats
Mulberries
Non-dairy milk
  (coconut, hemp,
  flax, almond)

Oatmeal
Okra
Onions
Oranges
Prunes
Pumpkin seeds
Rhubarb
Salmon
Sardines
Sesame seeds
Spinach
Tahini
Turnip greens

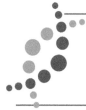

"Humans are the only species on earth that drink another mammal's milk and the only species that drinks milk after it has completed breast feeding."

Gluten

Over the past few years the word gluten has become so popular. Gluten is a protein found in wheat, rye, and barley including other grains related to wheat. For many people it is very difficult to digest. Foods that contain gluten are inflammatory foods and are also acidic forming in the body. Some people do not have the ability to digest gluten causing an immune response which damages the lining of the small intestine. This is known as celiac disease causing an interference of the body's ability to absorb nutrients. This lack of absorption can lead to bone disease and anemia. More commonly are those with gluten sensitivity otherwise known as wheat intolerance.

Gluten is found in many more products today than in years past due to the increase in processed foods. The growing of wheat has also changed over the years. In the past, it took many months to grow wheat – tall and golden. Today wheat as with many other ancient grains grows rapidly and is cultivated to produce more food on less land. The result is a crop with much higher levels of gluten.

So how do you know if you have sensitivity to gluten? Symptoms can vary for each individual and can include abdominal pain, bloating, diarrhea and/or constipation, a skin rash, joint or bone pain, fatigue and depression. If you suspect intolerance, remove gluten from the diet for a few weeks (elimination diet) to see if symptoms improve. If there is sensitivity, removing gluten from the diet can create health benefits specifically for the athlete – increased energy and better sleep.

Gluten can be found in many products and even places that you wouldn't expect.

"Good nutrition will prevent 95% of all disease."
~Linus Pauling

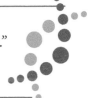

Where does gluten hide?

Alcoholic drinks (beer, ale, lager)
Baked beans
Biscuits or cookies
Bread and bread rolls
Some breakfast cereals (All Bran, Muesli)
Brown rice syrup
Cakes
Couscous
Crumble toppings
Gravy powder or bouillon cubes
Luncheon meats
Muffins
Pancakes and waffles
Pasta
Pastries and pie crusts
Pizza
Potato chips and pretzels
Salad dressings
Sauces
Soy sauce (Tamari is okay)

So what foods don't have gluten?

Whole fruits and vegetables, legumes, brown rice, quinoa, buckwheat, wild rice and oats. There are some flours used in baking that also do not contain gluten such as garbanzo (my favorite), brown rice, coconut, almond, hemp seed, millet and buckwheat. To get wholesome nutrition and gluten free options, eating great grains can provide that much needed source. These grains are absorbed into the system more slowly than refined grains helping to prevent spikes in sugar and insulin.

Great Grains

- ☑ Brown rice
- ☑ Buckwheat
- ☑ Oats, steel cut
- ☑ Quinoa
- ☑ Wild rice
- ☑ Popcorn (organic)
- ☑ Cornmeal (organic)
- ☑ Amaranth

Please understand when a food is labeled "gluten-free" it doesn't necessarily mean it is any better for you. The "gluten-free" fad has become a breeding ground for companies to market their sub-par foods as healthy ones with a few key master marketing words such as "gluten-free". Often times, gluten-free products have added fat and sugars to make them palatable which can easily increase the calorie amount. Avoiding highly processed foods will lead to a healthier and happier digestive system.

If you're at the store and still not sure if gluten is in the product, just look for foods that have but one ingredient. Eating whole foods is always the right option.

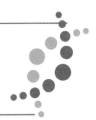

"When a food is labeled 'gluten-free' it doesn't necessarily mean it is any better for you."

Sugar and Artificial Sweeteners

Natural sugars found in fruit are essential for your survival and for optimum athletic performance. However a majority of today's packaged and processed foods are infested with chemically made refined sugars. These are extremely unnatural to the human body and most of these refined sugars are derivatives of GMO corn or beets. The combination of the refined sugars and the incredibly high amounts being consumed has created an epidemic of disease and illness across the globe, especially here in North America. The food industry has become extremely savvy by constantly changing the names of the sugars they use in their processed foods so that people don't even realize what they are eating. They also do a good job of sneaking in three or four different types of sugars so "sugar" doesn't top the list of ingredients in food labels. A good portion of today's processed foods contain unnecessary amounts of **sugar** and are "hidden" on labels under different names. *(See next page)*

Athletes in particular must be religiously consuming the proper types of sugar to maintain the highest level of performance and to maintain that sustained energy which will help avoid the "crash" and a drop in performance. Foods like dates are high in glucose, and upon consumption act as instant energy as the glucose is rapidly converted to glycogen in the liver. For sustained energy it is an absolute must to maintain a proper glycogen supply in both the muscles and the liver.

Fructose derived from fruit is also key for sustained performance because of its slow release. Agave nectar is a natural sweetener that comes from the blue agave cactus and is an exceptional choice for athletes or anyone engaging in any type of exercise because it consists of 90% fructose. A combination of dates and agave nectar are near perfect for all athletic performance and are extremely easy to consume prior and during competition.

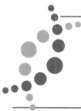

"A low-glycemic menu is chock full of fiber and protein. Low-glycemic foods encourage a slow and steady digestion so you feel fuller longer."

Sugar by Another Name

Agave nectar
Barley malt
Beet sugar
Blackstrap molasses
Brown-rice syrup
Brown sugar
Cane sugar
Cane juice crystals
Caramel
Carob syrup
Castor sugar
Coconut palm sugar
Confectioner's sugar
Corn sweetener
Corn syrup or corn syrup solids
Crystalline fructose
Date sugar
Dehydrated cane juice
Demerara sugar
Dextrin
Dextrose
Diastatic malt
Diatase
D-mannose
Dried oat syrup
Evaporated cane sugar
Fructose
Fruit juice concentrate

Galactose
Glucose
Golden syrup
Gum syrup
High fructose corn syrup
    (HFCS)
Honey
Invert sugar
Lactose
Maltodextrin
Malt syrup
Maltose
Mannitol
Maple syrup
Molasses
Palm sugar
Raw sugar
Rice syrup
Saccharose
Simple syrup
Sorbitol
Sorghum or sorghum
    syrup
Sucrose
Syrup
Table sugar
Treacle
Turbinado syrup
Xylose

When reading labels, typically those ingredients ending in "ose" or "ol" are more than likely sugars.

The amount of sugar in a product can be determined by looking at the number of grams in the item. Four (4) grams of sugar equals one (1) tsp. For example, if the label states that there are 20 grams of sugar in the item, that equates into five (5) teaspoons. The daily maximum amount of sugar from all sources should be no more than 36 grams for men and 20 grams for women.

Also hidden on labels in processed foods are **artificial sweeteners** under different names as well.

Acesulfame-K
Alitame
Aspartame
Aspartame-acesulfame salt
Cyclamates
Isomalt
Neotame
NutraSweet
Saccharin
Splenda
Sucralose

Glycemic Index

Next, we need to look at where the ingredient falls on the **glycemic index**. **Glycemic index** is a measure of how a food influences blood glucose after the food has been eaten. A low-glycemic menu is chock full of fiber and protein. Low-glycemic foods encourage a slow and steady digestion so you feel fuller longer.

Low GI

Artichokes and artichoke hearts
Asparagus
Bamboo shoots
Beans:
  Green
  Kidney
  Garbanzo
Bean sprouts
Berries:
  Blackberries
  Blueberries
  Boysenberries
Cucumber
Daikon Radish
Eggplant
Greens:
  Collard
  Kale
  Mustard
  Turnip
Leeks
Lentils
Mushrooms
Okra

Low GI *(continued)*

Elderberries
Gooseberries
Loganberries
Raspberries
Strawberries
Broccoli
Brussels sprouts
Cabbage:
  Green
  Bok choy
  Chinese
Cauliflower
Celery

Onions
Pea pods
Peppers
Radishes
Rutabaga
Squash
Sugar snap peas
Swiss chard
Tomato
Watercress
Zucchini

Moderate GI

Apples
Avocados
Cherries
Fresh apricots
Grapefruit
Kiwi
Lemons
Limes
Melons
Nectarines

Oranges
Passion fruit
Peaches
Pear
Persimmons
Plums
Pomegranates
Tangerines

The higher the glycemic index, the greater the spike in blood glucose. Up and down spikes in blood sugar are to be avoided.

High GI

Banana
Dried apricots
Grapes
Mango

Papaya
Pineapple
Raisins
Watermelon

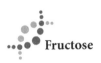 **Fructose**

Fruit	Serving Size	Grams of Fructose
Lime	1 medium	0
Lemon	1 medium	0.6
Cranberries	1 cup	0.7
Passion fruit	1 medium	0.9
Prune	1 medium	1.2
Guava	2 medium	2.2
Date	1 medium	2.6
Cantaloupe	⅛ of medium melon	2.8
Raspberries	1 cup	3.0
Clementine	1 medium	3.4
Kiwi	1 medium	3.4
Blackberries	1 cup	3.5
Star fruit	1 medium	3.6
Cherries, sweet	10	3.8
Strawberries	1 cup	3.8
Cherries, sour	1 cup	4.0
Pineapple	1 slice (3.5" x 0.75")	4.0
Grapefruit, red or pink	½ medium	4.3
Boysenberries	1 cup	4.6
Tangerine/ mandarin orange	1 medium	4.8
Nectarine	1 medium	5.4
Peach	1 medium	5.9
Orange (navel)	1 medium	6.1
Papaya	½ medium	6.3
Honeydew	⅛ of medium melon	6.7
Banana	1 medium	7.1
Blueberries	1 cup	7.4
Date (Medjool)	1 medium	7.7

Fruit	Serving Size	Grams of Fructose
Apple	1 medium	9.5
Persimmon	1 medium	10.6
Watermelon	1/16 medium melon	11.3
Pear	1 medium	11.8
Raisins	¼ cup	12.3
Grapes, seedless (red or green)	1 cup	12.4
Mango	½ medium	16.2
Apricots, dried	1 cup	16.4
Figs, dried	1 cup	23.0

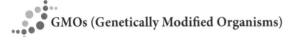

GMOs (Genetically Modified Organisms)

Also known as Genetic Engineering (GE) or Genetic Modification (GM) of food, this process takes place in the laboratory where genes are artificially inserted into the DNA of food crops or animals creating combinations that do not occur in nature. The outcome of this process is a genetically modified organism (GMO). Consuming GMOs may create an ill effect on the body, and may also cause damage to the environment. GMOs can be engineered with genes from viruses, insects, bacteria, animals, and humans and have never been proven to be safe for human consumption. Labeling of such products is absolutely necessary as we consumers need to know what's in the food we are purchasing. Unfortunately, here in North America food and beverage companies are not required to properly label GMO ingredients, which is why many processed foods contain these cheap, subsidized ingredients like corn, soy and canola.

Strategies to avoid GMOs

☑ Buy organic – Those foods that are certified organic are not permitted to contain any GMOs. Look for labels that read "100% organic," "organic," or "made with organic ingredients" to assure you are purchasing a non-GMO product. If an item is labeled "made with organic ingredients," then only 70% of the ingredients are organic but 100% must be non-GMO.

☒ Avoid products made with GM ingredients – typically used in processed foods, GM ingredients consist of corn, soy, canola, cottonseed and sugar.

Corn – Corn meal, flour, oil, gluten and syrup; sweeteners (fructose, dextrose and glucose); modified food starch.

Soy – Soy lecithin, protein, flour, isolate and isoflavone.

Canola – Canola oil also known as rapeseed oil.

Cottonseed – Cottonseed oil.

Sugar – Beet sugar.

☑ Buy products labeled "NON-GMO" Some companies have begun to label products "NON-GMO" or "Made Without Genetically Modified Ingredients" voluntarily. Reading the entire label will insure you are actually purchasing the product intended.

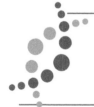

"GMO presents a certain unquantifiable risk, since there's a lot we don't know about these crops."
~ **Michael Pollan**

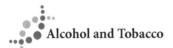# Alcohol and Tobacco

Alcohol

You need a healthy liver to process toxins from your body and to metabolize fats. However, the consumption of alcohol causes your liver to go into overdrive to work harder to rid of the accumulated toxins, prevents new glucose from being formed, and causes muscle repair to be diminished.

While society fully embraces alcohol in all its forms, what effect does it really have on overall health and performance? The most obvious side effect with the consumption of alcohol is that it dehydrates the body. It is a powerful diuretic that can cause severe dehydration and extreme electrolyte imbalances. Severe dehydration can require several days to a week for full recovery. A dehydrated athlete is at a much greater risk for muscle strains, cramping, and musculoskeletal injuries and puts your brain at a higher risk for a possible concussion. Dehydration can also lead to a decrease in appetite and a loss of muscle mass which results in a decrease in strength and performance. Whether you drink beer, wine or mixed drinks, it can all have detrimental effects on both the quality and duration of sleep and also on daytime attention. Since sleep is an essential part of the recovery process, the disruptive nature of alcohol interferes with both deep sleep and REM sleep, not allowing your body to fully recover and be well rested. Lack of sleep can have repercussions on daytime performance. Even several days after consumption, alcohol can impair reaction time and mental acuity, leading to a possible decrease in hand-eye coordination and impaired judgment. Alcohol also interferes with lactic acid breakdown and can result in decreased energy, decreased muscle recovery, and increased muscle soreness.

Alcohol creates an acidic environment in your body and overstimulates cells in the lining of the stomach that produce acid. Increases in acid production are associated with heartburn and ulcer development. Intestinal cells fail to absorb micronutrients (vitamins and minerals), which can lead to more electrolyte imbalances and vitamin deficiencies. This can weaken your immune system, causing your body's natural defense system to be operating below optimum levels. In this state, your body may be more vulnerable to sickness and infection. For anyone trying to shed a few pounds, alcohol isn't the help you are looking for. Alcohol has seven calories per gram.

Fat has nine calories per gram. Alcohol is stored much like fat in the body and even destroys amino acids and stores them as fat that ultimately leads to an increase in body fat. Alcohol, when consumed in amounts typical with binge drinkers, can dramatically decrease serum testosterone levels which can lead to a decrease in muscle recovery, lean muscle mass and overall athletic performance.

Long-term alcohol use may lead to weakened heart muscle, impotency, altered brain and nerve functions, elevated triglycerides, fat deposits in the liver, abnormalities in blood-clotting, pancreatitis, liver failure and other vitamin deficiencies. Besides the negative side effects alcohol has on general health and performance, it is often the main ingredient in many current social problems we see today such as domestic disputes, fatal auto accidents, and fights resulting in injury or incarceration.

Alcohol has ruined the lives and careers of many an athlete in one way or another. It is a powerful substance and it needs to be respected. Don't let this get in the way of reaching your goals and living out your dreams. While it is pretty obvious that alcohol can prevent one individual from reaching their ultimate playing potential, it can also have a very negative impact on the whole team concept. The team is only as good as the sum of its parts and if some of the parts aren't on their game it can mean the difference in winning and losing and ultimately the difference between being a champion or not.

The facts mentioned above are not shared to scare you but to make you more aware. Alcohol decreases performance and increases your risk of injury. Although it may not be realistic to eliminate the use of alcohol altogether, intensive efforts should be made in this direction because of the detrimental side effects listed previously. If you are going to have a drink or two, be sure to mix in a water or coconut water between drinks and before bed to help prevent any dehydration. Drink responsibly. Drink consciously.

Tobacco
Chewing tobacco, also known as smokeless tobacco, is no better than smoking a cigarette. The nicotine is just as addictive and can cause tooth decay and heart disease. Chewing tobacco has also been known to cause a variety of cancers including lip, tongue, mouth, pharynx, esophageal, and pancreatic.

With chewing tobacco come discolored teeth. A natural way to improve the staining is by "oil pulling". Oil pulling is quick and easy to incorporate into your morning routine. Before stepping into the shower, take one tablespoon of coconut or sesame oil and begin to swish it around in your mouth between your teeth, over your tongue, and your gums all the while showering for 5 to 20 minutes. The oil will become frothy and white. Do not swallow the oil or gargle with it. Upon getting out of the shower, spit all the oil out. Thoroughly rinse your mouth and brush your teeth as you normally would. Repeat this process daily.

Another good practice is brushing and flossing your teeth twice daily. You want to look for toothpastes that do NOT contain Triclosan as this was first registered as a pesticide in 1969 and now is widely used as an anti-microbial. Triclosan, when combined with water forms chloroform, a possible carcinogen. And when exposed to sunlight, triclosan forms dioxins which are known endocrine disruptors.

If you have difficulty or find it cost prohibitive to buy toothpaste without Triclosan, consider making your own. This recipe is easy, tasty and non-expensive.

Homemade Toothpaste
Combine equal parts coconut oil and baking soda (6 tablespoons each).

Add therapeutic grade essential oil(s) to taste (15 drops).
Cinnamon – anti-fungal, anti-bacterial, anti-viral, anti-oxidant
Clove – anti-viral, anti-bacterial, anti-fungal, anti-oxidant
      (may kill candida)
Eucalyptus – anti-fungal, anti-bacterial, anti-viral, anti-inflammatory
Lemon – anti-fungal, anti-bacterial, anti-viral, anti-inflammatory,
      anti-oxidant
Orange – anti-oxidant, anti-septic
Peppermint – anti-oxidant
Rosemary – anti-fungal, anti-bacterial, anti-viral

Combine and store in a glass jar by the bathroom sink.

"Long-term alcohol use may lead to weakened heart muscle, impotency, altered brain and nerve functions, elevated triglycerides, fat deposits in the liver, abnormalities in blood-clotting, pancreatitis, liver failure and other vitamin deficiencies."

Body Balance in Review – Part Three

☑ Inflammation can wreak havoc on your body causing numerous health problems along the way. A clean and nutrient dense diet consisting of anti-inflammatory foods will lead toward your body's natural ability to heal.

☑ Being awake for hours or waking throughout the night creates stress on the body. It's important to find balance for a restful night's sleep which consists of a variety of strategies.

☑ There are pros and cons to caffeine. Learn what works best for you to balance your body.

☑ Dairy products are not the only way to get calcium, and Vitamin D and more. There are a variety of foods that work together naturally to give you the nutrients you need.

☑ From gluten sensitivities to full blown celiac disease, inflammation is at the forefront here. So many processed products may contain hidden sources of gluten causing a variety of symptoms.

☑ Natural sugars from fruit are essential for your survival and for optimum athletic performance. Sugar found in processed and packaged products, however, are unnatural to the body.

☑ A handy listing of fruits with serving size and fructose content to help you choose your daily intake wisely.

☑ Labeling of Genetically Modified Organisms is necessary for you, the consumer, to know what you are putting into your body making the best decisions for health and wellness.

☑ Alcohol consumption and tobacco use causes numerous negative effects on the body and performance.

> *"Alcohol can be the cause of poor quality sleep, abdominal issues, added fat calories causing weight gain, and decreased performance on the ice.*

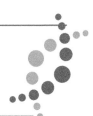

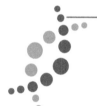

"Being a conscious eater is simply doing your best with the options you have."

Part Four

Does A Body Good

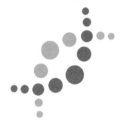

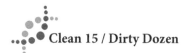 **Clean 15 / Dirty Dozen**

Being a conscious eater is simply doing your best with the options you have. Some foods are naturally cleaner than others whether they are organic or not. Sometimes an organic produce option might not be available or is just too expensive. The list of the **Clean 15 and Dirty Dozen** foods below are resources provided by the Environmental Working Group (EWG) (http://www.ewg.org). Their mission is to protect public health and the environment. In doing so, EWG has specialized in providing up-to-date information to you, the consumer, on such topics as "Skin Deep" and "EWG's Shopper's Guide to Pesticides." EWG is a non-profit organization founded in 1993.

The **Clean 15** vegetables and fruits are those that do not necessarily need to be purchased organically. These items have minimal pesticide residues with 7% of the samples having just one pesticide detected.

1. Avocados
2. Corn
3. Pineapples
4. Cabbage
5. Sweet peas - frozen
6. Onions
7. Asparagus
8. Mangoes
9. Papayas
10. Kiwi
11. Eggplant
12. Grapefruit
13. Cantaloupe
14. Cauliflower
15. Sweet potatoes

The **Dirty Dozen** consist of those vegetables and fruits which are the most contaminated by pesticides. When purchasing these produce items, it is of utmost importance to buy organic. (This listing has been expanded by EWG to be more inclusive).

1. Apples
2. Strawberries
3. Grapes
4. Celery
5. Peaches
6. Spinach
7. Sweet bell peppers
8. Nectarines – imported
9. Cucumbers
10. Cherry tomatoes
11. Snap peas - imported
12. Potatoes
13. Hot peppers +
14. Kale/collard greens +

To receive a full listing, you can download the information at the app store. It's very handy especially when you're at the grocery store.

"Keeping your body healthy is an expression of gratitude to the whole cosmos — the trees, the clouds, everything."
~ **Thich Nhat Hanh**

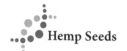 **Hemp Seeds**

The nutritional profile of the hemp seed is so impressive that it is often referred to as the "perfect food." Hemp seed/or nut is the most nutritious and easily digestible food on the planet. It is the only complete source of plant-based protein, essential amino acids (for cellular detoxification, production of vital enzymes, and muscle growth and repair) and essential fatty acids (EFA). These tiny seeds are a great source of fuel for everyone, athlete or not. In fact the hemp seed is the only food on earth that supplies all man's dietary needs in one food source meaning that it is the only food which can sustain human life without any other source of nutrition.

The hemp seed is jam packed with nutrition. It is made up of approximately 44% healthy edible fats. Roughly 81% of these fats are unsaturated "good fats" that are made up of essential fatty acids (EFAs). Hemp seed oil contains all EFAs and delivers the highest amount of EFAs of any plant on earth. Hemp oil has been labeled "Nature's most perfectly balanced oil" due to its perfectly balanced 3.75:1 ratio of Omega 6 (linoleic/LA) to Omega 3 (alpha-linolenic/LNA).

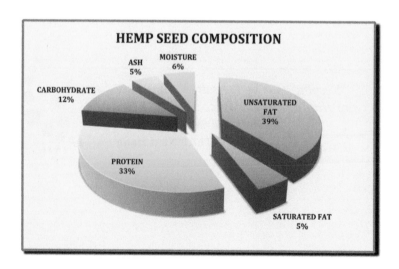

The EFAs in hemp seeds help battle inflammation due their powerful anti-inflammatory properties. It is also an excellent source of the LA derivative super-polyunsaturated Gamma Linolenic Acid (GLA) at 2.5-3% of volume which is only found in a handful of natural foods.

Omega fatty acids are EFAs. Your body does not produce them so they need to be ingested through your nutrition. These fats do not raise cholesterol levels, in fact they help clear the body's arteries. The healing properties in EFAs help general health and well being, maintain hormonal balance, and create healthy skin and hair. A deficiency of these fats has been linked to many diseases such as cancer, cardiovascular disease, autoimmune disorders, multiple sclerosis, skin and hair disorders, and more.

Hemp seeds contain an unusually high amount of plant-based protein. Approximately 33% of the seed is protein and is second only to soy (35%) but is much more digestible because 65% of the protein in hemp seeds is made up of the globulin protein Edestin. Edestin helps create healthy digestion. This nutritional powerhouse is a complete protein and contains 20 amino acids including all 10 essential amino acids. This is extremely instrumental in muscle and tissue regeneration for athletes.

Hemp protein is alkaline forming and is extremely digestible therefore making it a **ENERGY** + food. Hemp seeds contain chlorophyll, vitamin E, important B vitamins, folic acid as well as essential minerals including calcium, magnesium, phosphorus, potassium, sulfur and iron. They are involved in energy metabolism, protein and bone synthesis, and have trace elements that maximize oxygen levels. Hemp seeds are also high in dietary fiber and contain twice the protein found in flax seeds and chia seeds. Hemp seeds are naturally non-GMO.

For the athlete, hemp can calm post-workout inflammation as hemp foods have anti-inflammatory properties and help relax tense muscles making it the perfect post-workout snack. (see Recipes)

Fiber

Fiber is an extremely important part of the foods you consume as it aids in the digestion process. On average, you should aim for approximately 32 grams of fiber daily. For women, that would be 21-25 grams per day and for men 30-38 grams per day. Some research even says you should be consuming up to 50 grams of fiber daily.

If fiber has not been a consistent part of your daily nutrition, don't try to increase it too rapidly. Too fast of an increase can lead to gas, bloating, diarrhea, constipation, and an overall sense of not feeling well. Gradually increase fiber by adding more whole foods and less processed foods to your diet.

Many foods contain both soluble and insoluble fiber. Soluble fiber helps slow the release of carbohydrates into the bloodstream which controls insulin levels and ultimately prolongs energy levels. Soluble fiber makes you feel full. The role of insoluble fiber is to ensure a healthy digestive track by controlling and cleaning out toxins so they do not build up and spread into the bloodstream.

Foods that are higher in fiber consist of berries and fruit (apples and oranges), nuts (almonds and pistachios), seeds (chia seeds or freshly ground flax seeds), beans (lentils, black beans and split peas), and non-starchy vegetables (broccoli and Brussels sprouts). (see High-Fiber Foods for a more detailed list). Foods that are not fiber dense are meats, dairy products and refined grains.

But what is fiber exactly? Fiber is that part of a plant-based food your body is not able to digest. These foods are rich in water which helps to keep you feeling full longer. Fiber also helps in slowing down digestion, and moving fat through the digestive system causing less fat to be absorbed. Fiber supports the gut by providing good bacteria, decreasing bad bacteria, aids in maintaining proper pH, boosts the immune system and allows your body to absorb much needed nutrients, and balances blood sugar.

When you increase fiber in your daily nutrition, make sure to also increase water. Water helps to move food through the digestive system creating positive results as listed above.

If you are having issues with constipation, consider increasing fiber sources by approximately 5 grams daily. Supplements to choose from are:

☑ Psyllium husks help in moving yeast and fungus out of the body, and are used in managing cholesterol.

☑ Brown rice bran is high in fiber, vitamins, minerals, antioxidants, and essential fatty acids with a mild, nutty flavor.

☑ Chia seeds are high in antioxidants, anti-inflammatory, and a great source of omega-3 fatty acids and calcium. When combined with water, they form a gel-like consistency with a poppy-seed taste.

"Fiber is that part of a plant-based food
your body is not able to digest."

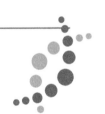

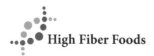 **High Fiber Foods**

Fruits	Serving Size	Total fiber (grams)*
Apple, with skin	1 medium	4.4
Banana	1 medium	3.1
Figs, dried	2 medium	1.6
Orange	1 medium	3.1
Pear, with skin	1 medium	5.5
Raisins	1 ounce (60)	1.0
Raspberries	1 cup	8.0
Strawberries	1 cup (halves)	3.0
Grains, cereal and pasta		
Barley, pearled, cooked	1 cup	6.0
Bran flakes	¾ cup	5.3
Bread, rye, whole-wheat, multigrain	1 slice	1.9
Brown rice, cooked	1 cup	3.5
Oat bran muffin	1 medium	5.2
Oatmeal, cooked	1 cup	4.0
Popcorn, air-popped	3 cups	3.5
Spaghetti, whole wheat, cooked	1 cup	6.3

Fiber content can vary between brands

Legumes, nuts and seeds	Serving Size	Total fiber (grams)*
Almonds	1 ounce (23 nuts)	3.5
Black beans, cooked	1 cup	15.0
Hemp seeds	3 Tbsp.	3.0
Lentils, cooked	1 cup	15.6
Lima beans, cooked	1 cup	13.2
Pecans	1 ounce (19 nuts)	2.7
Pistachio nuts	1 ounce (49 nuts)	2.9
Split peas, cooked	1 cup	16.3
Sunflower seed Kernels	¼ cup	3.9

Vegetables (steamed, cooked or as noted)

Artichoke	1 medium	10.3
Broccoli	1 cup	5.1
Brussels sprouts	1 cup	4.1
Carrot, raw	1 medium	1.7
Green peas	1 cup	8.8
Potato, w/skin, baked	1 small	3.0
Sweet corn	1 cup	4.0
Tomato paste	¼ cup	2.7
Turnip greens	1 cup	5.0

Fiber content can vary between brands

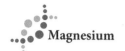 **Magnesium**

Magnesium is one of those extraordinary nutrients found in our bones, muscles, blood, and other tissues. It is the fourth most abundant mineral found in cells after calcium, phosphorus and potassium. Magnesium is needed by our bodies to synthesize fat and protein, produce energy, relax muscles, metabolize calcium, and operate the nervous system. Maintaining a sufficient amount of magnesium is necessary to balance blood sugar, decrease muscle cramps, alleviate migraine headaches, anxiety, reduce heart palpitations and the dangers of heart disease, strengthen bones, and delay the process of aging.

Too many of us are magnesium deficient as we do not take in the amount necessary to maintain a healthy body. Additionally, magnesium deficiencies can occur due to stress, whether that stress is physical or emotional, and can occur from taking certain medications such as diuretics, for example. Drinking too much coffee has a diuretic effect on the body again creating a deficiency.

Let's look at specific issues associated with low magnesium levels:

☑ Musculoskeletal – muscle soreness (back, neck, tension, headache), muscle cramps, muscle tension, painful spasms, twitching, poor muscle function and strength, restless leg syndrome

☑ Digestive – constipation, difficulty swallowing

☑ Metabolic – insulin resistance, carbohydrate intolerance, low serum calcium and potassium, elevated serum phosphorus, Vitamin D resistance

☑ Psychological – anxiety, depression, irritability, panic attacks

☑ Cardiovascular – arrhythmia (irregular heartbeat), palpitations, hypertension (high blood pressure), cardiac arrest, sudden death

☑ Pulmonary – asthma, allergic reactions, cold air triggers, bronchitis

☑ Neurologic – sinus and migraine headache, numbness and tingling, ringing in the ears, vertigo, hearing loss, insomnia

☑ Genitourinary – urinary spasm, kidney stone

☑ Other – carbohydrate, salt and chocolate cravings

It is recommended that a blood test for magnesium be checked to determine if a supplement would be necessary. Typically, multivitamins do not contain a sufficient amount of magnesium. If a magnesium supplement is needed, it should be combined with calcium.

Let's look at some of the benefits magnesium brings to our health and wellness.

☑ Musculoskeletal – muscle cramp relief, increased energy, increased muscle strength, improved structural support as in bone health when combined with calcium

☑ Psychological – as a muscle relaxant reducing muscle tension. Magnesium activates the making of GABA (gamma amino butyric acid) allowing for mental relaxation

☑ Cardiovascular – reduces heart palpitations, decreased risk for sudden cardiac death, relaxation of blood vessel walls that may aid in blood pressure

☑ Metabolic – improved insulin resistance, improved fasting blood sugar, improved blood pressure

☑ Neurologic – improved nerve pain, decrease in headache (migraine, cluster)

☑ Pulmonary – decreased asthma/allergy triggers

There are numerous foods that contain magnesium but most people do not get enough in their daily nutrition. It is estimated that 80% of the population is deficient. The following list contains foods rich in magnesium.

Food Sources	Amount	Magnesium (mg)	Calories
Almonds	1 oz.	78	164
Artichokes (hearts), *cooked*	½ cup	50	42
Beet greens, *cooked*	½ cup	49	19
Black beans, *cooked*	½ cup	60	114
Bran ready-to-eat cereal 100%	1 oz.	103	74
Brazil nuts	1 oz.	107	186
Brown rice, *cooked*	½ cup	42	108
Buckwheat groats, *roasted, cooked*	½ cup	43	78
Buckwheat flour	¼ cup	75	101
Bulgur, *dry*	¼ cup	57	120
Cashews, *dry roasted*	1 oz.	74	163
Cowpeas, *cooked*	½ cup	46	100
Great northern beans, *cooked*	½ cup	44	104
Haddock, *cooked*	3 oz.	42	95

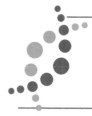

"Magnesium deficiencies can occur due to stress, whether that stress is physical or emotional, and can occur from taking certain medications such as diuretics, for example."

Food Sources	Amount	Magnesium (mg)	Calories
Halibut, *cooked*	3 oz.	91	119
Hazelnuts	1 oz.	46	178
Lima beans, baby, *cooked from frozen*	½ cup	50	95
Navy beans, *cooked*	½ cup	48	127
Oat bran, *raw*	¼ cup	55	58
Okra, *cooked from frozen*	½ cup	47	26
Oat bran, *cooked*	½ cup	44	44
Peanuts, *dry roasted*	1 oz.	50	166
Pine nuts, *dried*	1 oz.	71	191
Pollock, walleye, *cooked*	3 oz.	62	96
Pumpkin & squash seed kernels, *roasted*	1 oz.	151	148
Quinoa, *dry*	¼ cup	89	159
Spinach, *cooked from fresh*	½ cup	78	20
Tuna, yellowfin, *cooked*	3 oz.	54	118

"My kitchen is my Wellness Center."

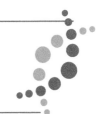

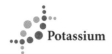 **Potassium**

Potassium is an important electrolyte as it is essential in cellular function. Potassium boosts immunity and energy levels, protects the heart, helps to lower blood pressure, and improves digestion. Most importantly for the athlete, potassium helps maintain fluid balance, builds muscle and strengthens bones. The average daily intake of potassium for an adult is 4,700 milligrams.

Foods Rich in Potassium

1,000 mg

Baked potato – 1-8 ounce with skin on

Beet greens – ¾ cup, cooked

Edamame – 1 cup shelled, cooked (preferably organic)

Halibut – 4 ounce

Lima beans – 1 cup, cooked

White beans – 1 cup (canned – rinse well and drained)

750 mg

Papaya – 1 large

Plantains – 1 cup, cooked

Sweet potato – 1 cup, cooked

Tomato sauce – 1 cup

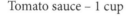

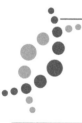

"Potassium is a vital mineral, which helps normalize the heartbeat, send oxygen to the brain and regulates your body's water balance. When we are stressed, our metabolic rate rises, thereby reducing our potassium levels."

500 mg

Apricots, dried – 12 halves

Avocado – ½ medium

Banana – 1 large

Beets – 1 cup, cooked

Cantaloupe – 1 cup

Mushrooms – 1 cup, cooked

Prunes – 9

Salmon – 4 ounces

Squash, winter – 1 cup, cooked

250-350 mg

Celery – 1 cup, raw

Chicken, breast – 5 ounces, roasted

Kiwi – 1 medium

Mango – 1

Nectarine – 1

Orange – 1 medium

Peanut butter – 2 Tbsp.

Peanuts – 1 ounce or ¼ cup

Pear – 1 large

Raisins – ¼ cup

Red bell peppers – 1 cup

Squash summer – 1 cup, raw

Strawberries – 1 cup (preferably organic)

Watermelon – 1 wedge

Zinc

Zinc is an essential mineral necessary in creating DNA, maintaining a healthy level of enzymes, supporting a sense of smell, decreasing inflammation, and healing the gut. Zinc deficiencies can lead to nausea, diarrhea, vomiting, abdominal discomfort, headache and decreased appetite. Zinc deficiencies can occur as zinc is depleted in the soil from farming processing and distribution. A minimum of 15 mg. is recommended daily and 30 mg. for vegetarians. If necessary, consider taking zinc acetate, zinc glycinate or gluconate to boost levels.

Foods Rich in Zinc

- ☑ Beans – cooked mung beans, baked beans, adzuki beans, lentils, garbanzo beans
- ☑ Beef and Lamb
- ☑ Mushrooms – cooked white mushrooms, raw morel, brown and white, dried and raw shitake
- ☑ Quinoa
- ☑ Seafood – cooked oysters, crab, lobster
- ☑ Sesame seeds
- ☑ Spinach
- ☑ Wheat Germ

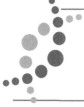

"Zinc is essential to your health, boosting the immune system, helping cells to grow, regulating appetite and healing wounds."

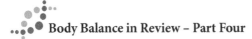 **Body Balance in Review – Part Four**

☑ When purchasing foods, having the most up-to-date information is necessary to make the best possible choices when it comes to clean foods.

☑ The most digestible protein, rich in essential fatty acids and fiber, hemp is a fuel source for athletes and non-athlete's alike. Superfood!

☑ Fiber aids the digestive process and keeps us feeling fuller longer.

☑ This listing of high fiber foods provides a variety of food sources consisting of serving size and total grams of fiber to help you choose and boost your daily intake.

☑ Magnesium is one of those nutrients vital for energy. It decreases muscle cramps, strengthen bones, aids in sleep, and more.

☑ Potassium helps maintain fluid balance which is especially important for the athlete.

☑ Another mineral, zinc, is important in helping to decrease inflammation and heal the gut.

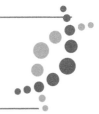

"The most digestible protein, rich in essential fatty acids and fiber, hemp is a fuel source for athletes and non-athlete's alike. Superfood!"

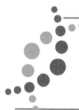

"Let the food be thy medicine and thy medicine be thy food."

~ **Hippocrates**

Part Five

Recipes

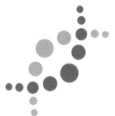

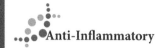 **Anti-Inflammatory**

Anti-inflammatory Turmeric Tea

Ingredients:

1 cup non-dairy milk (almond, hemp)
½ tsp. turmeric
1 tsp. cinnamon
1 tsp. raw honey
¼ tsp. ginger

Directions:

Heat the milk slowly in a small pot on the stove.
Stir in the spices and drizzle the honey on top.
Great after an evening game before bed.

Anti-inflammatory Green Smoothie

Ingredients:

1 cup fresh or frozen pineapple
1 handful arugula
1 handful kale and spinach
½ inch fresh ginger root, peeled
1-½ cups coconut water and/or green tea
½ tsp. turmeric powder or ½ inch fresh turmeric
   root
½ tsp. cinnamon
1 scoop protein powder of choice (optional)

Directions:

Blend all ingredients. Top with chia seeds or
hemp seeds, and walnuts or almonds.

Anti-Inflammatory Tonic

Ingredients:

1-½ cups pure water
⅓ cup fresh lemon juice
1 tsp. turmeric or ½ tsp. freshly grated turmeric
Dash of cinnamon
1 Tbsp. maple syrup

Directions:

Pour water into glass. Add remaining ingredients, and stir.

Anti-Inflammatory Turmeric Dip

Ingredients:

1 cup raw cashews, soaked overnight, drain
1 Tbsp. olive or hemp oil
1 cloves garlic
¼ cup coconut milk
1 Tbsp. turmeric
1 tsp. ground ginger
1 Tbsp. raw honey

Directions:

Add above ingredients to food processor or
high-speed blender. Blend until smooth. Serve
with raw vegetables of choice (carrots, cucumber,
celery, broccoli, cauliflower, etc.).

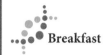 **Breakfast**

Porridge

Ingredients:

½ cup oats or quinoa
1 cup water
1 Tbsp. flax, chia and/or hemp seed
½ tsp. cinnamon
1 Tbsp. currants

Directions:

Mix all ingredients in a saucepan and cook until
water is absorbed.

Pumpkin Pie Oatmeal

Ingredients:

½ cup oats
½ cup mashed pumpkin or ½ can pumpkin puree
½ cup coconut milk
1 cup water
1 tsp. vanilla extract
1 tsp. pumpkin pie spice
1 Tbsp. maple syrup or raw honey

Directions:

Mix all ingredients in a saucepan. Cook until
liquid is absorbed.

Rice Porridge with Apples

Ingredients:

2 cups leftover brown rice or quinoa with ¼ cup
    water, coconut water, or desired non-dairy milk
1 Tbsp. maple syrup
1 tsp. ground cinnamon
Pinch of sea salt
1 apple, peeled and diced

Directions:

Add rice, liquid, maple syrup, cinnamon and
salt to pan and cook over medium low heat.
Add apple and mix well. Bring mixture to a boil,
then reduce heat to low and simmer. Continue
cooking for about 10 minutes or until the apple
is soft.
Yield: 3 servings

Protein Packed Porridge

Ingredients:

1 cup non-dairy milk of choice
1 tsp. almond butter
1 tsp. maple syrup or raw honey
½ tsp. cinnamon
½ tsp. vanilla extract
¼ tsp. cardamom
3 Tbsp. chia seeds
½ cup fresh fruit of choice
Walnuts, almonds (if desired), to taste
Coconut (if desired), to taste

Directions:

Heat first 6 ingredients over medium heat until
heated through but not boiling (for 3-5 minutes).
Mix in chia seeds, remove from heat and let
mixture sit for 10 minutes, stirring occasionally.
Top with fruit. Additionally, top with nuts of
choice and coconut, if desired.

Granola #1

Ingredients:

2 cups oats
1 cup mixed raw nuts
¼ - ½ cup mixed seeds (sunflower, chia, pumpkin,
   poppy, hemp, sesame, flax)
¾ cup unsweetened shredded coconut
1 tsp. cinnamon
5 Tbsp. pure maple syrup
3 Tbsp. olive or coconut oil
1-½ cups dried fruit

Directions:

Preheat oven to 350° F. Combine oats, seeds,
coconut and cinnamon, and put on baking sheet.
Stir well and smooth out. Drizzle syrup and oil
over all; stir. Bake 25-30 minutes checking every
5 minutes. When mixture is slightly browned,
remove from oven, and mix in dried fruit. Cool
completely and store in an airtight jar. Stores up
to 2 weeks.

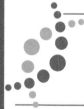

*"Oats gain part of their distinctive flavor
from the roasting process that they undergo
after being harvested and cleaned."*

Granola #2

Ingredients:

2 cups oats
5 Tbsp. coconut oil
1 tsp. cinnamon
1 tsp. ginger
½ cup pumpkin seeds
½ cup sunflower seeds
1 cup shredded, unsweetened coconut
1 cup raw almonds
½ cup walnuts
2 Tbsp. raw honey

Directions:

Mix all ingredients together, spread on a lipped
baking sheet. Bake at 160° F for 20 minutes,
stirring half way through, until crunchy.

*"Virgin (or unrefined) coconut oil has a very
light, sweet-nutty coconut flavor and aroma.
Refined coconut oil is basically tasteless."*

Oatmeal Pancake *(also great for a post-workout meal)*

Ingredients:

¼ cup oats
2 eggs
¼ tsp. baking powder (aluminum-free)
¼ tsp. cinnamon
¼ tsp. vanilla extract
Pinch salt
1 Tbsp. water
½ banana, mashed or applesauce
Toppings:
Fruit (raspberries, blueberries, strawberries)
Dried fruit (raisins, unsweetened cranberries)
Nuts (almonds, walnuts)
Seeds (hemp seeds, chia seeds)

Directions:

Combine ingredients together and cook like a
pancake. Top with assorted toppings.

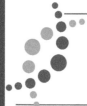

*"Oatmeal pancakes are quick and tasty
and a delicious way to entice your family
into eating healthy."*

Burgers

Lentil Burgers

Ingredients:

3 cups water
2 cups lentils
2 cloves garlic, minced
½ cup fresh cilantro, finely chopped
2 Tbsp. tamari soy sauce
1 Tbsp. olive oil
1 Tbsp. umeboshi vinegar
1 medium onion, chopped

Directions:

Bring water to a boil. Add lentils, reduce heat to simmer and cook uncovered for 40 minutes until lentils become soft and loose their shape. While lentils are cooking, sauté onion and garlic in olive oil until translucent. Remove from heat and set aside with remaining ingredients. Preheat oven to 400° F. When lentils are finished, transfer to a large mixing bowl and cool in freezer for 10 minutes. Remove from freezer and add all other ingredients and mix well. Form into patties, 4 inches in diameter and ¾-inch thick. Place patties on a lightly oiled cookie sheet and bake 10-15 minutes in the oven.

Prep Time: 10 minutes
Cooking Time: 1 hour
Yields: 8 servings

Sweet Potato Burgers

Ingredients:

1-2 large sweet potatoes, baked, peeled and mashed
   to equal about 2 cups
2-15 oz. cans white cannellini beans (drained and
   rinsed well)
2 Tbsp. tahini
2 tsp. maple syrup
1 tsp. Cajun seasoning
¼ cup flour (brown rice, oat, garbanzo, etc.)
"Bread" crumbs (Panko, gluten–free, brown rice,
   etc.)
Optional: Additional seasoning (dash or 2 of
cayenne, a scoop of nutritional yeast, salt and
pepper to taste)

Directions:

Bake sweet potatoes until fork tender. Allow to
cool, remove skin and place in a large bowl.
Combine sweet potatoes with beans and mash
together. Mash in seasonings and flour. Mixture
will be soft and moist. Thicken mixture if needed
with additional flour, crumbs or nutritional yeast.
Mold into patties and coat lightly with "bread"
crumbs.Bake in 350° F oven for 10-15 minutes.
May also cook in pan if desired.

*All burgers can be served on "bun" of choice. My
favorite "bun" is a large leaf of romaine! Top with
tomato, avocado, onion, pepper, Dijon mustard…
your choice of a variety of healthy toppings.*

Veggie Burgers

Ingredients:

2 cans black beans (rinsed and drained), mashed
½ cup uncooked quinoa – cooked to 1-½ cups
½ onion, minced
1 bell pepper, diced
2 tsp. cumin
2 eggs
"Bread" crumbs (Panko, gluten–free, brown rice, etc.)

Directions:

Mix all ingredients. Mold into patties. Cook on top of stove or bake at 350° F for 10-15 minutes.

"My favorite 'bun' is a large leaf of romaine!"

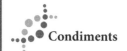 **Condiments**

Coconut Yogurt

Ingredients:

2 cups young coconut meal (from either opening a young coconut OR in the freezer section of an Asian market)

¼ cup coconut water, kefired water, or filtered water

¼ tsp. loose probiotic powder or from two probiotic capsules

Directions:

Add all ingredients to blender or food processor. Process until smooth and creamy, adding more coconut water until desired consistency is reached. Pour yogurt into a quart size mason jar. Allow enough room for expansion as it will grow by at least ⅓ volume. Cover and lightly tighten the lid in place. Put the jar in a bowl as the contents may over-flow, and place in a warm spot. Can be set in the oven with the oven light just barely on at 90° F for approximately 6-12 hours. Remove from warm area and carefully open in the bowl as over-flow may occur. Stir and store in the refrigerator lasting at least one week.

Ketchup

Ingredients:

1-6 oz. can (BPA free) tomato paste (no sugar added)
1-15 oz. can (BPA free) tomato sauce (no sugar added, low sodium)
1 tsp. onion powder
⅛ cup raw honey
Salt to taste

Directions:

Whisk all ingredients together until smooth. Place in fridge overnight giving flavors time to blend together.

This version is tasty, vegetarian and gluten free.

"Most bottled ketchup contains large amounts of sugar adding to the body's inflammation."

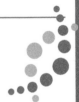

Mayonnaise

Ingredients:

½ cup raw cashews, soaked
2 Tbsp. lemon juice
1 tsp. honey or maple syrup
1 Tbsp. apple cider vinegar
2 Tbsp. pure water
¼ tsp. sea salt
½ cup olive oil

Directions:

Blend well drizzling the oil in last. Keeps in the refrigerator up to three weeks in a salad glass jar.

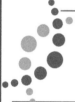

"Magnesium is the fourth most abundant mineral in the human body and is extremely important for healthy bones, muscles and nerves as well as for the heart and healthy blood sugar levels."

Dessert

Peanut Butter Banana Cookies

Ingredients:

2 cups oats
2 ripe bananas, mashed
½ cup nut butter of choice
¼ cup raw honey
1 cup unsweetened applesauce
½ cup raisins
½ cup chopped nuts of choice
2 Tbsp. flax seed, ground
1 Tbsp. cinnamon
1 Tbsp. vanilla extract

Directions:

Preheat oven to 350° F. Combine all ingredients.
Drop by the spoonful onto a parchment lined
baking sheet. Bake 20-30 minutes.

"Life is uncertain. Eat dessert first."
~ **Ernestine Ulmer**

Pudding

Ingredients:

2 cups non-dairy milk
4 Tbsp. chia seeds
1 medium banana, mashed
½ cup unsweetened shredded coconut
1 tsp. vanilla extract
1 Tbsp. maple syrup or raw honey
Garnish:
Berries
Mint leaves

Directions:

Place milk and chia seeds in a saucepan over medium heat and bring to a simmer, stirring occasionally with a whisk. When the mixture begins to thicken, whisk in remaining ingredients (except garnish), and simmer for 5-10 minutes, stirring occasionally. Divide mixture into 4 serving dishes and cool in refrigerator until firm, at least 1 hour. Garnish with berries and mint leaves.

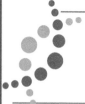

"Chia seeds are loaded with nutrients that have important benefits for your body and brain."

Entrees

Eggplant "Meatballs"

Ingredients:

1 medium eggplant, unpeeled and cut into 1" cubes
3-4 Tbsp. olive oil
1 medium onion, chopped
3-4 cloves garlic, minced
1 cup cooked or canned (drained and rinsed)
  white beans
¼ cup parsley, chopped
 Salt and pepper to taste
1 cup "bread" crumbs (choose from variety of whole
  grain, brown rice, etc.)
¼ tsp. red pepper flakes (optional)
Red sauce of choice

Directions:

Heat oven to 375° F. Grease a large rimmed
baking sheet with 1 Tbsp. oil. Heat 1 Tbsp. of oil
in a large pan over medium heat. When warm,
add the eggplant and ¼ cup water with salt and
pepper. Cook, stirring occasionally, until the
eggplant softens, 10 to 15 minutes. Transfer
to food processor or heavy duty blender. Add
1 Tbsp. oil to same pan along with onion and
garlic. Cook, stirring frequently, until onion
softens about 3-5 minutes.
Add beans and parsley to food processor with
the eggplant. Pulse until well-combined but not
pureed. Combine the eggplant mixture with the
onions and garlic. Blend in "bread" crumbs and
red pepper flakes, if desired. Roll mixture into
balls approximately 2 inches in diameter and
place on prepared baking sheet. Bake until firm
and browned 25 to 30 minutes. While "meatballs"
are baking, prepare red sauce of choice. Serve
with sauce over your choice of pasta, spaghetti
squash, spiralized zucchini, bed of greens, brown
rice or quinoa.

Easy Pasta Sauce

Ingredients:

2 Tbsp. olive oil
1 onion, chopped
2-3 cloves garlic, minced
2 broccoli crowns, cut into bite size pieces
8 ounces sliced mushrooms

Directions:

Heat the oil in a large pan over medium heat. Add garlic and onion; sauté to soften. Add broccoli and mushrooms. Continue to cook, stirring, until broccoli turns a bright green and the mushrooms soften. Toss with favorite cooked pasta, and serve.

"Pesto" Pasta

Ingredients:

4 cups spinach
1 cup fresh cilantro
2 - 4 cloves garlic to taste
6 sundried tomatoes
⅛ cup hemp seed
¼ cup olive oil
½ tsp. red pepper flakes
Juice of ½ lemon
Sea salt to taste
3 small zucchini spiralized or peeled into pasta-like strips

Directions:

Prepare zucchini as desired. In food processor or high speed blender combine remaining ingredients except olive oil. Start food processor or blender and add olive oil while blending. Mix "pesto" into zucchini "pasta."

Quinoa with Spinach and Garbanzos

Ingredients:

1 cup quinoa
2-¼ cups water or vegetable stock
Pinch of salt
1 medium onion, chopped
1 Tbsp. olive or coconut oil
½ cup dried cherries or cranberries (unsweetened)
1 bunch baby spinach (or green of choice)
1 cup garbanzo beans, cooked or canned (rinse and
    drain well)
Juice and zest from 2 oranges (preferably organic)

Directions:

Rinse quinoa and lightly toast in a dry pan a
few minutes until it smells nutty. Bring water or
stock to a boil; add salt and quinoa. Turn heat
to low and bring to a simmer, covered for 20
minutes or when all water is absorbed. Heat oil
in pan and sauté onions until translucent. Add
cherries, garbanzo beans, and spinach. Cover and
gently heat 3 to 5 minutes until spinach is wilted.
Remove from heat. Add cooked quinoa, orange
juice and zest. Stir gently and serve.

*"Quinoa is a good source of magnesium
and phosphorus, and is also
anti-inflammatory."*

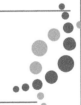

Hemp

Hemp Hummus

Ingredients:

1-½ cups chick peas (pre-soaked and cooked until soft)
4 Tbsp. hemp seeds
1 Tbsp. hemp or flax oil
1 tsp. garlic powder
⅓ cup lemon juice
½ tsp. salt
2 Tbsp. tahini (sesame paste)

Directions:

Place all ingredients in a food processor or high speed blender and mix until a creamy texture forms. Serve with raw veggies.

Hemp Protein Shake

Ingredients:

1 scoop of organic hemp protein powder
1 Tbsp. almond butter
1 cup almond milk or hemp milk
½ banana (preferably frozen)
3-5 ice cubes

Directions:

Combine all ingredients. Blend well.

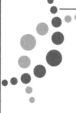

"Hemp seed is nutritious and contains more essential fatty acids than any other source, is second only to soybeans in complete protein (but is more digestible by humans), is high in B-vitamins, and is a good source of dietary fiber. Hemp seed is not psychoactive and cannot be used as a drug."

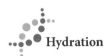 **Hydration**

Detox Water #1

Ingredients:

4 cups pure water
1 medium cucumber, sliced
1 lemon, sliced
Juice from 1 lemon
10-12 mint leaves
1 inch piece of ginger

Directions:

Steep overnight in fridge and drink daily. Great for general detoxification including clear skin.

Detox Water #2

Ingredients:

1 Tbsp. apple cider vinegar
1 Tbsp. lemon juice
1 tsp. cinnamon
Dash cayenne pepper
8 oz. pure water

Directions:

Mix well. Chill and serve.

Healthy Electrolyte Drink

Ingredients:

4 cups pure warm water
Juice of 1 lemon
2 tsp. honey
¼ tsp. salt

Directions:

Mix well. Chill and serve.

Prep Time: 2 minutes
Yields: 4 servings

Healthy Electrolyte Drink II

Ingredients:

8 oz. pure water
½ tsp. sea salt
½ tsp. baking soda
Lemon juice
1 tsp. maple syrup

Directions:

Mix well. Chill and serve.

Prep Time: 2 minutes
Yields: 1 serving

Switchel

Ingredients:

2 quarts pure water
½ cup apple cider vinegar
1/8 – ¼ cup raw honey
4 slices fresh, peeled ginger

Directions:

Combine in a pitcher or large jar.

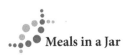 **Meals in a Jar**

Overnight Oats in a Jar

Ingredients:

⅓ cup oats
½ banana
⅓ cup plain yogurt of choice (see Condiments for
    Coconut Yogurt recipe)
⅓ – ½ cup non-dairy milk
¼ tsp. cinnamon
¾ Tbsp. chia seeds
Toppings:
Maple syrup
Small handful of almonds or walnuts
Nut butter
Cocoa powder or cacao nibs

Directions:

Mash banana in a bowl. Stir in oats, yogurt, milk,
cinnamon and chia seed. Mix until combined.
Place in a jar, cover and store in fridge overnight.
In the morning, top with maple syrup, nuts, and
any additional toppings of choice.

*"Apple cider vinegar may help in lowering
blood sugar, is a potent antimicrobial,
increases satiety, is a probiotic, and may
benefit the heart."*

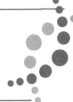

Porridge in a Jar (for breakfast or snack)

Ingredients:

¼ cup oat groats, rinsed and drained
¼ cup steel or rolled oats
1 tsp. currants
Sprinkle of cinnamon
4 oz. unsweetened almond milk (or other non-dairy milk)
1 tsp. chia seeds
1 cup fresh or frozen fruit of your choice

Directions:

In a glass jar of your choice, layer first 6 ingredients. Top with fresh or frozen fruit. Store in fridge over night or up to 3 days. Stir and enjoy cold right out of the fridge, at room temperature, or warmed in the oven for 10-15 minutes at 300° F.

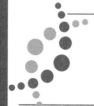

"Oats are a good source of dietary fiber."

Pudding in a Jar

Ingredients:

2-2-½ cups unsweetened almond, coconut or other
non-dairy milk of choice
½ cup chia seeds (full of omega-3 fatty acids,
calcium and fiber)
2-3 Tbsp. raw honey (optional)
½ tsp. vanilla extract (optional)
½ cup fresh or frozen fruit (raspberries,
blueberries, mango)
2 Tbsp. shredded coconut (optional topping)

Directions:

Combine above ingredients in a mason jar.
Shake well and place in refrigerator. Shake again
after half an hour. Refrigerate overnight or at
least 6 hours. The mixture will become thick
and pudding like. Divide equally into individual
servings and top with blueberries, raspberries,
mango or whatever fruit is available. Top with
coconut.

*"Pudding is a favorite dessert, snack or
treat for many people."*

Salad in a Jar

Ingredients:

Dressing
Almonds, arugula, beans, bell peppers, broccoli, carrots, chickpeas, cucumber, edemame, green beans, mixed greens, mushrooms, peas, quinoa, radishes, seeds, spinach, sprouts, strawberries, tomatoes, walnuts

Directions:

Bottom layer: dressing

Hearty Layer: beans, bell peppers, carrots, chickpeas, cucumber, edemame, green beans, radishes

Lighter layer: cooked quinoa, seeds, walnuts, sprouts, tomatoes, peas, mushrooms, broccoli, strawberries, almonds

Top Layer: lettuce, spinach, arugula, mixed greens

Enjoy as a snack or lunch.

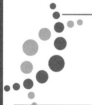

"Making one simple diet change, can pay off with plenty of health benefits."

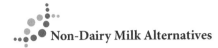 **Non-Dairy Milk Alternatives**

Almond Milk

Ingredients:

1 cup almonds soaked for 7 hours
3 cups pure water
3 dates or 1 Tbsp. honey (optional)
1 tsp. vanilla extract (optional)

Directions:

Pop the almonds out of their skins. Add all ingredients to the blender. Blend until smooth and milky. Strain in a nut strainer. Can use any kind of nut for this milk.

Yields: 3 cups of almond milk

Hemp Milk

Ingredients:

1 cup hemp seeds
3 cups pure water
3 dates or 1 Tbsp. honey (optional)
1 tsp. vanilla extract (optional)

Directions:

Add all ingredients to the blender. Blend until smooth and milky. Store milk(s) covered in the refrigerator for 4-7 days. Shake before serving.

Yields: 3 cups of hemp milk

For chocolate milk: add 1 tsp. cocoa powder
For strawberry milk: add ½ cup organic strawberries

Anti-Inflammatory Tumeric Milk

Ingredients:

2 cups non-dairy milk (rice, almond, hemp, coconut, or other nut milk)
1 tsp. turmeric
2 tsp. freshly grated ginger, or 1 tsp. ground ginger
½ tsp. ground cinnamon
¼ tsp. ground cardamom (optional)
2 pitted medjool dates or 1 Tbsp. maple syrup

Directions:

Blend all ingredients together in a blender Transfer mixture to a small pot and gently heat, stirring frequently. Serve warm.

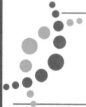

"Tumeric imparts an intense flavor, color, and distinctive fragrance to any recipe."

Salads

Quinoa Tabbouleh

Ingredients:

1 cup cooked quinoa (see below)
4 (or to taste) cherry tomatoes
2 or 3 (or to taste) scallions, or ¼ small yellow
   onion – can also use red onion
2 Tbsp. olive oil
4 squirts (or to taste) lemon juice
Salt and pepper to taste
Chopped parsley and/or basil to taste

Directions:

Chop veggies finely and add all other ingredients
together including cooked quinoa. Chill in
refrigerator, though not essential. Serve.

How to cook Quinoa: Use quinoa in ratio of 1:2
as in 1 cup quinoa to 2 cups water. Bring to a boil
and simmer 15 minutes. Quinoa expands to four
times its volume.

*"Quinoa is a quick-cooking, gluten free
whole grain grown in a rainbow of colors,
with the most common colors being red,
black and white."*

Quinoa, Broccoli and Chickpea Salad

Ingredients:

1 Tbsp. olive or hemp oil
1 small onion
2 tsp. fresh thyme, chopped
1 cup dry quinoa
2 cups pure water
2 cans chickpeas, drained and rinsed
1 head of broccoli cut into bite-size pieces and steamed
¼ cup fresh basil, chopped

Dressing:

2 -3 tsp. olive or hemp oil
¼ cup lemon juice (to taste)
Lemon zest (to taste)

Directions:

Heat oil over low heat in a large saucepan. Sauté onions until translucent with the thyme. Add dry quinoa and brown slightly. Add the water and bring to a boil. Reduce heat to a simmer, cover and cook for 15 minutes or until the water is absorbed. Toss quinoa mixture with the chickpeas, broccoli, and dressing. Add basil last, combine and serve.

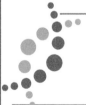

"While many people think of chickpeas as being beige in color, other varieties feature colors such as black, green, red and brown"

Bean Salad

Ingredients:

30 oz. canned black beans, rinsed well
30 oz. canned chickpeas, rinsed well
½ red onion, chopped
2-3 cloves garlic, minced
1 avocado, chopped
1 package grape tomatoes, halved
3 Tbsp. olive oil
2 Tbsp. cumin
Juice of 1 lime
Handful of cilantro

Directions:

Whisk together olive oil, cumin and lime juice in a large bowl. Add rinsed and drained beans and mix to combine. Add the onions, garlic avocado and cilantro. Mix well. Add more lime juice/olive oil to taste. Refrigerate.

"Brazil, along with India, grows more black beans than any country in the world."

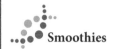 **Smoothies**

"After Workout" Smoothie

Ingredients:

1 cup unsweetened non-dairy milk (almond, hemp)
½ frozen banana
1 handful of spinach
1-2 kale leaves
1 Tbsp. almond butter
1 Tbsp. hemp seeds
1-2 Tbsp. goji berries
½ tsp. vanilla
½ - 1 tsp. cinnamon

Directions:

Combine all in a blender. Blend until smooth and serve.

"After Workout" Smoothie II

Ingredients:

1-2 frozen bananas
1 Tbsp. nut butter (almond, cashew – your choice)
1-½ cups unsweetened non-dairy milk
Additional Options:
Protein powder
Raw cacao
Flax seed
Chia seed
Hemp seed
Cinnamon

Directions:

Combine all in a blender. Blend until smooth and serve.

Carrot "Cake" Smoothie

Ingredients:

½ cup non-dairy milk (almond, coconut, hemp)
½ banana
1 small carrot, chopped
½ tsp. cinnamon
¼ tsp. nutmeg
¼ tsp. ginger
¼ tsp. cloves
1 tsp. ground flaxseed
1-½ tsp. shredded coconut
Ice cubes
Chopped walnuts

Directions:

Combine all in a blender. except walnuts. Blend until smooth. Top with chopped walnuts and additional coconut, if desired, and serve.

"Smoothies can be an easy way to nourish your body with essential nutrients."

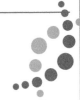

Green Smoothies are created with a variety of different items. When preparing your smoothies, aim for a 2-to-1 ratio of vegetables to fruit. Then you can add a variety of nutritional additions and a liquid. There are so many options in preparing a smoothie. Best thing to do – Experiment!! We all have different tastes, likes and dislikes. Pick what works best for you.

Leafy greens: spinach, kale, collards, bok choy, romaine and a variety of lettuces

Vegetables: celery, beets, pumpkin, cucumber, carrots, fennel

Fruit: berries, apple, banana, avocado, pineapple, mango, dates, pear and citrus

Liquids: pure water, coconut water, non-dairy milks (hemp, almond, coconut, oat), green tea

Nutritional additions: hemp seeds, chia seeds, flax seeds, protein powders, oats, nuts

Green Smoothie I

Ingredients:

1 avocado
1-2 pieces of a low glycemic fruit (green apple, pear, berries, cantaloupe)
1 cucumber
1 fistful of kale, spinach or romaine
Coconut water or purified water
Raw honey to taste, and/or sprinkle cinnamon or some cacao (optional)

Directions:

Prep and wash all produce. Blend until smooth and serve.

Green Smoothie II

Ingredients:

1 cup organic green veggie such as spinach, bok choy
½ large organic celery stalk
¼ cup parsley
½ organic cucumber
1 peeled lemon
½ - 1 banana
2 cups pure water

Directions:

Combine all in a blender. Blend until smooth and serve.

Hawaiian Smoothie

Ingredients:

1 cup chopped pineapple
1 frozen banana
½ cup unsweetened coconut water

Directions:

Combine all in a blender. Blend until smooth and serve.

Kiwi Kick Smoothie

Ingredients:

6 kiwis, peeled
6 celery stalks
1 pear

Directions:

Combine all in a blender. Blend until smooth and serve.

Power Smoothie

Ingredients:

2 cups almond, rice or hemp milk
1 cup fresh or frozen berries
½ cup frozen mango
2 Tbsp. almond butter
1 date, pitted
½ tsp. vanilla extract
Sprinkle of cinnamon
4-5 leaves kale
Handful of spinach

Directions:

Prep and wash all produce. Combine all in a blender. Blend until smooth and serve.

Powerful Protein Smoothie

Ingredients:

½ cup non-dairy milk of choice
1 cup spinach, kale or Swiss chard
1 stalk celery
Sliced cucumber
1 cup berries of choice
1 Tbsp. chia seeds

Directions:

Combine all in a blender. Blend until smooth and serve.

Vegan Muscle Building Smoothie

Ingredients:

Choose all organic if possible:
½ cup strawberries
¼ mango
½ frozen banana
½ cup green grapes
½ orange
2 kale leaves (stems removed)
½ cup oats
1 tsp. ground flax seed
1 cup cooled green tea
2 cups non-dairy milk of choice

Directions:

Combine all in a blender. Blend until smooth and serve.

Watermelon Smoothie

Ingredients:

Approximately 3 cups cubed, frozen watermelon
2-½ cups unsweetened non-dairy milk

Directions:

Combine all in a blender. Blend until smooth and serve.

"Watermelon is a nutrient dense food."

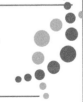

Snacks

Apple Chips

Ingredients:

2 apples, sliced crosswise ⅛-inch thick, seeds removed

Directions:

Heat oven to 225° F. Arrange apple slices on two parchment-lined baking sheets and bake for 1-½ hours. Flip, then continue baking until crisp, about 1 hour more. Remove and let cool completely. Chips keep, stored in an airtight container, 1 week.

Avocado Dip

Ingredients:

1 large peeled and pitted avocado
⅔ cup plain, goat or almond yogurt
1 diced tomato
Dash or 2 of cayenne pepper
Sea salt and black pepper to taste

Directions:

Mash avocado with a fork until very smooth. Add yogurt, tomato, and cayenne. Blend until smooth. Add sea salt and pepper to taste. Serve chilled with mixed raw veggies.
Best made approximately 1 hour before serving.

Cauliflower Hummus

Ingredients:

1 small head of cauliflower, chopped into pieces
1-2 cloves garlic
1 can chickpeas, drained and rinsed
1-2 Tbsp. tahini
1 Tbsp. olive oil
¼ cup scallions, chopped
¼ cup parsley
2 tsp. cumin
¼ tsp. paprika
3 Tbsp. lemon juice
⅛ cup pure water

Directions:

Cook cauliflower until soft. Drain and add remaining ingredients to food processor or high speed blender. Puree until smooth. Serve chilled with raw veggies.

Roasted Edamame

Ingredients:

1 bag organic shelled edamame (frozen)
1 Tbsp. olive oil or coconut oil
Sea salt to taste
Spices (turmeric, garlic…any spices you want)

Directions:

Place edamame in a bowl and drizzle with oil. Toss until evenly coated. Spread on a parchment lined baking sheet. Sprinkle with spices of choice. Bake at 375° F for 45 minutes stirring every 15 minutes.

Evening Snack

Ingredients:

1 small apple, sliced
Handful of pumpkin seeds

High in magnesium, aids in sleep

Frozen Treat

Ingredients:

1 ripe banana
1-2 Tbsp. roasted sunflower seeds, pumpkin seeds,
   chopped nuts (almond, walnuts)

Directions:

Roll peeled banana over seeds or nuts of choice.
Wrap in wax paper and freeze overnight. Cut into
slices and enjoy.

Guacamole

Ingredients:

2 ripe avocados
1 lime, juiced
2 medium cloves garlic, minced
¼ cup onions, chopped (optional)
½ cup tomatoes, chopped (optional)
Handful of cilantro
½ tsp. cumin
½ tsp. chili powder
¼ tsp black or white pepper
½ tsp. sea salt

Directions:

Combine all ingredients in a bowl. Spices can be
adjusted to your own preference. Can be stored
in the fridge for approximately 36 hours.

Pumpkin Spice Trail Mix

Ingredients:

1 cup oats
1 cup raw almonds
1 cup pecan halves
1 cup roasted shelled pumpkin seeds
1 cup walnut halves
¼ cup pumpkin puree
2 Tbsp. all natural apple juice
1-2 Tbsp. raw honey
⅔ cup dried cranberries
⅔ cup raisins
2 tsp. ground cinnamon
2 tsp. paprika
1 tsp. pumpkin pie spice

Directions:

Preheat oven to 250° F. Mix cinnamon, paprika and pumpkin pie spice in a bowl. Set aside. Place almonds, oats, pecans, pumpkin seeds, and walnuts in a bowl. Mix together pumpkin puree, apple juice and honey; pour over nuts and toss until evenly coated. Sprinkle nuts with spice mixture, tossing to coat well. Spread mixture evenly on 2 baking sheets. Bake 30-35 minutes, stirring halfway through cook time. Cool completely. Stir in cranberries and raisins. Store in an airtight container.

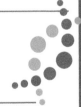

"Pumpkin is an often-overlooked source of fiber."

Kale Chips

Ingredients:

1 bunch kale, stems removed, broken into bite size pieces

Drizzle of olive oil, coconut oil, hemp oil

Seasoning options to taste:

Sea salt

Chili powder

Garlic powder

Cayenne pepper

Nutritional yeast

Directions:

Knead kale with oil of choice and seasoning(s) of choice. Bake in 250-300° F oven (checking every 5-10 minutes) until crispy.

Salsa:

Ingredients:

½ small yellow onion, chopped

1 clove garlic, chopped

1 small jalapeno, chopped

1-½ pounds plum tomato, chopped

1 tsp. vinegar

2 tsp. fresh oregano, chopped

¾ tsp. coarse salt

Directions:

In a food processor, pulse onion, garlic, jalapeno and ⅔ of the tomatoes until chopped. Transfer to a bowl. Pulse remaining ⅓ tomatoes until liquified. Add to bowl with vinegar, oregano and salt. Stir to combine.

Trail Mix

Ingredients:

2 cups almonds, raw
1 cup pecans
2 cups walnuts, raw
2 cups pumpkin or squash seed, raw
2 cups dried cranberries, unsweetened
1 Tbsp. olive oil or coconut oil (optional)

Directions:

In a bowl, mix together almonds, pecans, walnuts and seed. Cover with water and soak overnight. Preheat oven to 300° F. Rinse and discard soaking water. Add cranberries and oil. Mix until everything is coated well. Spread the mixture out evenly on baking sheet and place in oven for about 20 minutes or until you can smell the roasting nuts. Cool and store in air tight glass container. Try any nuts and dried fruit you like. The nuts and seeds do not have to be soaked or can be soaked for a few hours, but doing so helps their digestibility.

"Soaking nuts and seeds for a few hours will help with digestibility."

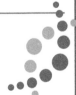

Raw Zucchini Hummus

Ingredients:

2 cups zucchini, cut into 1 inch pieces
⅓ cup lemon juice
¾ cup tahini
¼ cup olive oil
1 clove garlic
1 tsp. sea salt (to taste)
2 tsp. cumin

Directions:

Blend all ingredients in food processor or high speed blender until creamy and smooth. Serve with raw veggies.

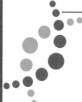

"Chia seeds are full of Omega-3 fatty acids, calcium and fiber."

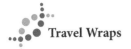 **Travel Wraps**

In preparing the following wraps, you can use romaine, collard or kale leaves removing the center stem if thickened. Green leaves will not get soggy like your wrap would if using tortillas.

Travel Wrap #1

Ingredients:

½ cup hummus
½ avocado, sliced
1 Tbsp. olives
1 Tbsp. raw sauerkraut
2 tsp. hemp oil

Directions:

Prepare two green leaves of choice.

Divide hummus spreading half on the center of each leaf. Top with remaining ingredients and wrap.

"Hummus is so rich in protein, it can help fight hunger cravings and balance blood sugar levels."

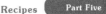

Travel Wrap #2

Ingredients:

1-15 oz. can chickpeas, drained and rinsed
½ red pepper, chopped
¼ cup fresh cilantro, chopped
¼ cup raisins
2 cups baby spinach

Dressing:

2 Tbsp. olive oil
½ tsp. raw honey
½ lime, juiced
1 tsp. curry powder
Salt and pepper to taste

Directions:

Prepare two green leaves of choice.

Mix together chickpeas, raisins, cilantro and red pepper in a large bowl. In a separate small bowl, combine dressing ingredients. Add dressing to the chickpea mixture and stir well. Divide the mixture between 2 large green leaves. Top with 1 cup each of baby spinach and wrap.

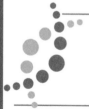

"Cilantro is very low in calories and contains no cholesterol."

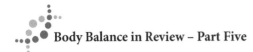

Body Balance in Review – Part Five

☑ My wish for you is to create your kitchen, your "Wellness Center", full of whole, nutrient dense foods.

> *"Make gradual, lifestyle changes to empower you to attain and support your current and future health goals."*

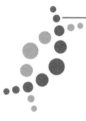

"I want to provide the needed information for you to make very educated decisions when it comes to the fuel you put into your body, your temple, and for you to dig deep into looking at your life style, what you are eating, and if it's working for you or against you."

~ **Deborah Dittner**

Resources

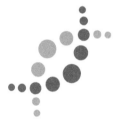

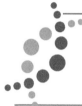

"Imagine how fantastic life would be if you had a balanced, healthy lifestyle that's exciting, nourishing and free of denial and deprivation."

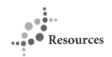

Resources

☑ http://www.The-Balanced-Body.com
The-Balanced-Body, created by Deborah Dittner, guides you toward creating optimal health with a holistic approach and lifestyle changes in health and wellness. Together, we will explore concerns specific to you and your body and discover the tools you need for a lifetime of balance.

☑ http://www.brendanbrazier.com
Brendan Brazier is a professional ironman triathlete, creator of VEGA, a whole food, plant- based nutritional product, and best-selling author on plant-based nutrition. His books include *Thrive Foods, Thrive Energy Cookbook, Thrive The Vegan Guide to Optimal Performance in Sports and Life* and more.

☑ http://www.deborahdittner.vibrantscents.com
Explore Therapeutic Grade Essential Oils offering natural remedies to life's imbalances. Essential oils, produced by Mother Nature, bring harmony to mind, body and spirit. Twenty years ago, D. Gary Young founded Young Living Essential Oils preserving the integrity and potency of natural essential oils. Young Living is committed to meeting specific criteria in four key areas: Plants, Preparation, Purity, and Potency.

☑ http://www.drinksoma.com
The Soma carafe was designed to make it simple to always have fresh filtered water on hand. The glass carafe is easy to hold, stored on the counter or refrigerated, and uses an all-natural filter made from coconut shell carbon and housed in a plant-based casing.

☑ http://www.drweil.com
Dr. Andrew Weil graduated from Harvard Medical School and has traveled the world studying healers and healing systems. He has authored numerous books earning the reputation as an expert on alternative medicine.

☑ http://www.EFTUniverse.com
Emotional Freedom Technique is a form of energy therapy with the intention to rebalance the energy system.

☑ http://www.eastcoastfloatspa.com
Flotation Therapy assists in decreasing inflammation in the joints, muscle and joint pain, and creating relaxation. This therapeutic approach has been popular in Europe and now is gaining attention here in the states.

☑ http://www.ewg.org
The mission of the Environmental Working Group (EWG) uses the power of public information to protect the health of the public and the environment. EWG specializes and provides the resources for the "EWG's Shopper's Guide to Pesticides" and "Skin Deep".

☑ http://www.hemphealsfoundation.com
The Hemp Heals Foundation, created by Riley Cote, supports sustainable agriculture and sustainable health while educating people on health and nutrition. Hemp, a nutrient rich superfood, is a highly digestible protein and fiber, high in essential fatty acids (EFAs), and has anti-inflammatory properties.

☑ http://www.integrativenutrition.com
The Institute for Integrative Nutrition (IIN), founded and directed by Joshua Rosenthal, is a school at the forefront of holistic nutrition education. IIN offers comprehensive training introducing a wide variety of dietary theories while enriching your mind, nurturing your body, and maximizing your health.

☑ http://www.jjvirgin.com
New York Times best-selling author, nutrition and fitness expert JJ Virgin discusses the 7 food intolerances and how changing your nutrition can change your life. Her books include *The Virgin Diet, The Virgin Diet Cookbook, Six Weeks to Sleeveless and Sexy* and more.

☑ http://www.kriscarr.com
Best-selling author and cancer survivor Kris Carr shares wellness tips and motivation for health and wellness. Her books include *Crazy Sexy Cancer Tips, Crazy Sexy Diet, Crazy Sexy Cookbook* and more.

☑ http://www.manitobaharvest.com
Manitoba Harvest is the world's largest hemp food manufacturer to grow, make and sell their own line of hemp foods. At Manitoba Harvest they strive for sustainability and educate on the health and environmental benefits of hemp.

☑ http://www.nutribullet.com
Nutrition and longevity expert, David Wolfe, uses the Nutribullet in his videos pertaining to superfood nutrition.

☑ http://www.nutritionstudies.org
Dr. T. Colin Campbell and the Center for Nutrition Studies. Dr. Campbell has been at the forefront of nutrition and health studies for over 40 years. Dr. Campbell has co-authored *The China Study: Startling Implications for Diet, Weight Loss and Long-term Health and Whole: Rethinking the Science of Nutrition.*

☑ http://www.teeccino.com
America's #1 coffee alternative with recipes and health tips for building optimal health.

☑ http://www.ultrawellnesscenter.com
The UltraWellness Center with founder and medical director Mark Hyman, MD, is located in Lenox, MA. Here you will find the key to lifelong health and vitality while learning about nutrition, mindfulness, exercise, stress management, sleep and more.

☑ http://www.vitamix.com/index.asp
For whole food nutrition, reducing waste, and saving time and money.

06-005616

GET FREE STANDARD SHIPPING ($25US/$35CN) USE ABOVE CODE

1-800-848-2649

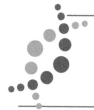

"When you smile, the whole world smiles with you!"

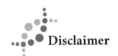

Disclaimer

The information provided in **Body Balance Empowering Performance** is for **education purposes only** and is in no way intended to replace the advice of your health care professional or any information contained on or in any product label or packaging.

You should not use the information featured in **Body Balance Empowering Performance** for diagnosis or treatment of any health condition or as a substitute for medication or other treatment prescribed by your health care professional.

The statements in **Body Balance Empowering Performance** have not been evaluated by the Food and Drug Administration.

Every individual is different, thus what may work for one may not work for another person. How you react to a particular product may be significantly different from the way another person may react to the same product.

Consult one-on-one with the health care professional of your choice.

Taking responsibility for your health is your own personal decision. I recommend that you continue to research and choose wisely in balancing your body for overall health and wellness.

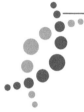

"*The mission here is quite simple. My vision is to help empower all people. Athlete or not, this book will help you look at things a bit differently and help guide you along in your journey no matter what it might be. My goal is to explain nutrition in the simplest way using basic common sense so you will all have the knowledge to consciously choose foods wisely.*"

~ **Deborah Dittner**

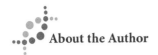 **About the Author**

Deborah Dittner, FNP-C, RMT, CHHC, AADP

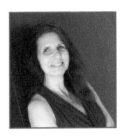

Deb received her BS in Nursing from Western Connecticut State University, her certificate as a Primary Care Nurse Practitioner from Albany Medical College, and Reiki Master Teacher certificates from the Reiki Room of Saratoga Springs, NY. She is a graduate of The Institute for Integrative Nutrition (IIN) in NYC in 2009, which combines the knowledge of traditional philosophies with modern concepts of different dietary theories. Deb continued at IIN through the Immersion program in 2010, 2011 and 2012 while counseling students enrolled in the professional training program. She has been honored in Marquis Who's Who in Medicine and Healthcare and has been affiliated with Saratoga Integrative Practitioner's Network (SIPN) since its inception.

Deb has been a longtime advocate and provider of integrative and holistic practices. She strongly believes in supporting men and women to improve their health and wellness through a variety of lifestyle changes including, but not limited to, high quality nutrition, physical activity, relationships, family, career and community. She will personalize your daily nutrition while exploring the necessary tools needed to create a lifetime of balance. Food changes everything. Imagine what your life would be like if you had clear thinking, energy, and excitement every day.

Deb has experience in family health, pediatrics, women's health, college health, athletics, and holistic counseling.

For more information, you can go to
http://www.The-Balanced-Body.com
or call 518-596-8565.

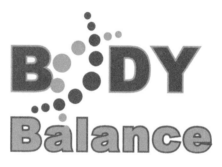

CPSIA information can be obtained at www.ICGtesting.com
Printed in the USA
BVOW11s1046021214

377497BV00008B/11/P